CHPN®

Practice Questions

Mometrix
TEST PREPARATION

Dear Future Exam Success Story

First of all, **THANK YOU** for purchasing Mometrix study materials!

Second, congratulations! You are one of the few determined test-takers who are committed to doing whatever it takes to excel on your exam. **You have come to the right place.** We developed these practice tests with one goal in mind: to deliver you the best possible approximation of the questions you will see on test day.

Standardized testing is one of the biggest obstacles on your road to success, which only increases the importance of doing well in the high-pressure, high-stakes environment of test day. Your results on this test could have a significant impact on your future, and these practice tests will give you the repetitions you need to build your familiarity and confidence with the test content and format to help you achieve your full potential on test day.

Your success is our success

We would love to hear from you! If you would like to share the story of your exam success or if you have any questions or comments in regard to our products, please contact us at **800-673-8175** or **support@mometrix.com**.

Thanks again for your business and we wish you continued success!

Sincerely,
The Mometrix Test Preparation Team

Written and edited by the Mometrix Exam Secrets Test Prep Team
Printed in the United States of America

TABLE OF CONTENTS

Practice Test #1

1. A 54-year-old patient with end-stage renal failure dies of sudden cardiac arrest 6 days after withdrawal of dialysis. This patient's death was most likely caused by which of the following complications of renal failure?

a. Hypercalcemia
b. Anemia
c. Hyperkalemia
d. Hyperphosphatemia

2. Which of the following is most accurate regarding poorly controlled pain in the palliative care patient?

a. Uncontrolled pain leads to multiple harmful physiological effects.
b. Inadequate treatment of pain usually enhances a patient's ability to interact with loved ones.
c. Uncontrolled pain only causes psychological harm to the patient.
d. Adequate pain control makes it more difficult to promptly identify complications of the patient's disease.

3. Which of the following statements is most appropriate regarding advanced care planning in the terminally ill patient?

a. Advanced care planning should address issues beyond code status.
b. The best time for advanced care planning discussions is late in the course of a terminal illness.
c. Advanced care planning decisions should be made after a single conversation.
d. Advanced care planning discussions are outside the scope of practice for the palliative care nurse.

4. Which of the following is most accurate about heat therapy for the treatment of pain?

a. Heat therapy is most effective for the treatment of neuropathic pain.
b. Application of heat results in decreased blood flow to the treatment area.
c. Heat therapy is highly effective for treatment of pain associated with muscle spasm.
d. Heat therapy is most effective over areas with decreased sensation.

5. A 50-year-old patient with metastatic ovarian cancer has been receiving home hospice care provided primarily by her partner and a home health aide. The patient's partner becomes unable to care for her, and the patient's condition worsens, so that she now requires at least 12 hours of active nursing care daily for symptom management. The patient's level of hospice service under the Medicare Hospice Benefit is best described as:

a. Routine home hospice care
b. Continuous home hospice care
c. General inpatient hospice care
d. Inpatient respite care

6. Among the following, the sign most likely to indicate that the hospice nurse is not maintaining appropriate professional boundaries with a patient or family is:

a. Believing that he or she is the only nurse that can take good care of the patient
b. Encouraging the patient's loved ones to say goodbye as death approaches
c. Crying at the bedside when the patient dies
d. Keeping in touch with a patient's family after the patient has died

7. The medical team caring for a terminally ill cancer patient is hesitant about broaching the topic of palliative care team consultation with the patient. Initial discussion of palliative care team consultation should include emphasis on all of the following EXCEPT:

a. Expertise of the palliative care team in managing the disease-related symptoms the patient is experiencing
b. Information the palliative care team can provide that helps ensure that the patient is fully informed about his or her choices
c. The expertise of the palliative care team in helping the patient maximize quality of life
d. The fact that there is nothing more the medical team can do for the patient

8. A colon cancer patient returns home after a colostomy, and the patient's wife tells the nurse, "I don't think I can change the colostomy bag as well as the nurses do." The nurse's best response is:

a. "You should have told me sooner if you didn't feel comfortable with this."
b. "Tell me how you learn best and we'll work together until you feel comfortable changing the colostomy bag."
c. "Watch me change the colostomy bag and let me know if you have any questions."
d. "Maybe it would be best if someone else in your family could take responsibility for changing the colostomy bag."

9. The palliative care nurse would expect all of the following symptoms in a patient with severe anemia EXCEPT:

a. Nosebleeds
b. Fatigue
c. Dyspnea
d. Pallor

10. A 70-year-old patient with advanced lung cancer is dyspneic despite sitting upright near a fan while receiving supplemental oxygen. The hospice nurse should:

a. Lay the patient flat.
b. Administer morphine.
c. Turn off the fan.
d. Administer glycopyrrolate.

11. Which of the following is most accurate about hypercalcemia in the setting of advanced malignancy?

a. Hypercalcemia in cancer patients is associated with poor prognosis.
b. Hypercalcemia is usually asymptomatic.
c. Bisphosphonate medications are contraindicated in the patient with hypercalcemia.
d. Hypercalcemia is rarely associated with breast cancer.

12. The first-line therapy for tumor-related brain edema is:

a. Anticonvulsants
b. Antibiotics
c. Mannitol
d. Steroids

13. Which of the following is most accurate regarding assessment of pain in the palliative care patient with limited cognition or communication ability?

a. Pain assessment is more dependent on nonverbal signs of discomfort.
b. Pain assessment scales cannot be used with these patients.
c. Family members are unreliable sources of information about pain in these patients.
d. Patients with cognitive deficits experience less pain than other patients.

14. Palliative ("terminal") sedation would be most appropriate for which of the following patients?

a. A 47-year-old breast cancer patient experiencing severe pain as an adverse effect of an experimental chemotherapeutic agent
b. A 27-year-old metastatic melanoma patient who wants to die "before things get bad"
c. A 54-year-old congestive heart failure patient with severe constipation due to opioid medications
d. A 69-year-old patient with advanced glioblastoma who has severe intractable headache despite maximal analgesic administration

15. Management of persistent hiccups in the palliative care patient may include all of the following EXCEPT:

a. Pharyngeal stimulation (e.g., palate massage)
b. Muscle relaxants (e.g., baclofen)
c. Decreasing gastric distention (e.g., smaller meals, gas agents)
d. Opioids

16. A patient with pharyngeal cancer whose plan of care involves only comfort measures develops acute, massive hemorrhage due to tumor erosion of the carotid artery. The hospice nurse should:

a. Ask the family to leave the room.
b. Apply a hemostatic dressing to the site of bleeding.
c. Administer blood products.
d. Provide supportive care to maximize patient comfort.

17. A patient has recently become sarcastic and sullen. When the hospice nurse asks if there is anything bothering him, he replies, "I'm angry, okay?" The nurse's best response is:

a. "It's not my fault that you're so sick."
b. "If you're willing, I'd like to hear more about what is making you angry."
c. "I know what you're going through."
d. "I can't help you until you're willing to be more respectful."

18. A palliative care patient with Alzheimer's dementia is wandering away from home while his family caregiver is sleeping. All of the following initial recommendations are appropriate in this case EXCEPT:

a. Install better locks and consider alarms on doors leading to exit routes.
b. Provide a secure place where the patient can wander safely.
c. Have the patient placed in a residential facility that is better equipped to manage Alzheimer's dementia.
d. Provide environmental visual cues to orient the patient within the home.

19. The nurse is caring for a 71-year-old Vietnamese patient with gastric cancer. Best practice for using an interpreter in the palliative care setting includes all of the following EXCEPT:

a. Speaking directly to the patient rather than the interpreter
b. Instructing the interpreter to simply repeat speech verbatim without offering additional cultural perspective
c. Using brief, clear statements without excessive medical jargon
d. Speaking with the interpreter before and after the patient interaction to ensure common understanding

20. A 47-year-old patient with amyotrophic lateral sclerosis (ALS) complains of nasal regurgitation of oral fluids and the sensation of solid food getting caught in her throat. This is most consistent with:

a. Xerostomia
b. Dysphagia
c. Gastroesophageal reflux
d. Aspiration pneumonia

21. Evaluation of a palliative care patient with suicidal ideation should include assessment of all of the following EXCEPT:

a. Details about the patient's specific suicide plan
b. Poorly controlled symptoms (e.g., pain) that are contributing to the patient's distress
c. The patient's mental status
d. State law regarding physician-assisted suicide in the terminally ill patient

22. The nurse is caring for a hospice patient who is on a continuous morphine infusion with as-needed bolus morphine doses for breakthrough pain. If the patient regularly requires several morphine bolus doses per hour for breakthrough pain, the most effective adjustment for improved pain control in this patient is:

a. Increase the basal morphine infusion rate.
b. Increase the bolus morphine breakthrough dose.
c. Add an adjuvant analgesic without changing morphine dosing.
d. Shorten the interval between bolus morphine breakthrough doses.

23. A hospice patient is being treated for constipation. Which of the following statements is most accurate regarding management of constipation in hospice patients?

a. Manual disimpaction is the therapy of choice.
b. Stool softeners and/or laxatives should be started with the initiation of opioid analgesics.
c. Oral fluid intake should be restricted in patients taking osmotic laxatives (e.g., lactulose).
d. Pharmacologic therapy is indicated only in patients with complications of constipation.

24. The wife of a patient with advanced lung cancer asks the nurse if her husband's fatigue, weight loss, and poor appetite mean he is depressed. The nurse should explain that:

a. Depression is appropriate in the terminally ill patient and does not require treatment.
b. Depression in terminally ill patients is defined by the presence of suicidal thoughts.
c. Physical symptoms of depression often overlap with symptoms of advanced cancer.
d. Depression is rare in the terminally ill patient.

25. A 34-year-old patient with advanced melanoma tells the hospice nurse that she feels guilty for "being such a burden" on her husband. The hospice nurse should:

a. Reassure the patient that caring for an ill wife is a husband's duty.
b. Discourage the patient from sharing her feelings with her husband.
c. Encourage the patient to express appreciation for the care her husband provides.
d. Encourage the patient to remind her husband how dependent she is on him now.

26. The hospice nurse is screening for caregiver stress in a patient's adult daughter. Which of the following is most concerning for a potentially unhelpful caregiver attitude?

a. The patient's daughter asks to be the only family member caring for the patient.
b. The patient's daughter is open to suggestions.
c. The patient's daughter expresses fear and uncertainty about the dying process.
d. The patient's daughter seeks out other resources in coping with her father's care.

27. Adults with cystic fibrosis most commonly die as a result of:

a. Sepsis
b. Pancreatic failure
c. Respiratory failure
d. Secondary malignancy

28. At which point is it most appropriate for the hospice nurse to discontinue routine vital sign monitoring in the palliative care patient?

a. Monitoring is interfering with the patient's end-of-life care preferences.
b. The patient has died.
c. The patient has refused artificial hydration.
d. The patient is no longer receiving any medications.

29. A 52-year-old patient with metastatic colorectal cancer complains of abdominal pain that he describes as "stretching and cramping." This is most consistent with:

a. Neuropathic pain
b. Visceral pain
c. Psychological pain
d. Somatic pain

30. Use of a fentanyl patch would be most appropriate in which of the following patients?

a. A 73-year-old lung cancer patient with severe, poorly controlled pain
b. A 26-year-old leukemia patient starting opioid therapy for bone pain
c. A 51-year-old hospice patient with severe pain associated with daily wound dressing changes
d. A 48-year-old melanoma patient with stable pain and dysphagia

31. A palliative care patient is complaining of bothersome pruritus. Management of pruritus in areas where skin is intact should include all of the following EXCEPT:

a. Identify and avoid exacerbating factors (e.g., heat).
b. Encourage scratching of affected areas.
c. Apply moisturizing creams/ointments.
d. Pat skin dry instead of rubbing.

32. A 55-year-old patient with anal cancer, whose death is expected in a matter of days, begins moaning, throwing off bed sheets, and experiencing apparent hallucinations. This is most accurately described as:

a. End-of-life pain
b. Dementia
c. Terminal restlessness
d. Complicated grief

33. The nurse is providing care to a home hospice patient as he dies. Supportive interventions for family members in the hours immediately after death should include all of the following EXCEPT:

a. Encourage loved ones to spend as much time with the deceased as they need to.
b. Bathe the patient before allowing the family to spend time with the deceased.
c. Assist the family with arranging transfer of the patient's body to the funeral home.
d. Remove medical equipment that is interfering with the family's ability to get close to the deceased.

34. A hospice patient develops progressive dyspnea that is improved with oxygen. As the nurse is preparing to teach the patient's son how to use the oxygen tank and mask, he says, "My girlfriend is a paramedic, so I already know how to use it." The nurse's best response is:

a. "Let's move on to something you feel less comfortable with."
b. "I doubt you have enough experience with this to care for someone as ill as your father."
c. "I still have to teach you about this anyway."
d. "Let's start with what you already know, and I can teach you what you need to know for making your dad most comfortable."

35. A patient with bladder cancer is taking sustained-release oral morphine twice daily for constant baseline pain. He consistently requires several doses daily of immediate-release oral morphine for adequate control of breakthrough pain and is experiencing no unpleasant adverse effects. The most appropriate pain management strategy with this patient is to:

a. Continue with the current analgesic regimen.
b. Increase the dosage amount of the immediate-release morphine.
c. Decrease the dosage interval of the immediate-release morphine.
d. Increase the dosage amount of the sustained-release morphine.

36. A hospice patient with multiple myeloma develops thirst, fatigue, constipation, and weakness. Among the following, the electrolyte abnormality most likely to explain these symptoms is:

a. Hypoglycemia
b. Hypercalcemia
c. Hyponatremia
d. Hypocalcemia

37. A 49-year-old hospice patient with a malignant wound complains about wound odor. Among the following, the most effective strategy for management of wound odor is:

a. Application of wet charcoal dressings
b. Less frequent dressing changes
c. Topical metronidazole to control anaerobic wound colonization
d. Application of silver nitrate–soaked gauze

38. A 61-year-old patient with lung cancer develops superior vena cava syndrome. On physical assessment of this patient, the nurse would expect to find:

a. Facial pallor
b. Flattened neck veins
c. Upper-extremity muscle wasting
d. Respiratory distress

39. The family of a patient who is new to the palliative care team asks the nurse what services are covered under the Medicare Hospice Benefit. All of the following are 100% covered without copay under the Medicare Hospice Benefit EXCEPT:

a. Family bereavement support after the patient's death
b. Durable medical equipment related to terminal illness
c. Nursing home room and board fees
d. Short-term inpatient care for symptom management

40. Comprehensive pain assessment of the palliative care patient is indicated in all of the following circumstances EXCEPT:

a. When the patient declines a pain assessment
b. After changes have been made in the pain management plan
c. When the patient reports a new type of pain
d. After administration of analgesic medication(s)

41. Which of the following routes of morphine administration will result in the shortest time to onset of analgesic effect?

a. Subcutaneous
b. Rectal
c. Intravenous (IV)
d. Oral

42. A patient with Alzheimer's dementia develops rapidly increasing confusion, increased heart rate, profound fatigue, and marked decrease in appetite over the course of 12 hours. This is most consistent with:

a. Impending death due to progression of disease
b. The expected waxing and waning course of Alzheimer's dementia
c. A potentially reversible cause of acute deterioration
d. The patient's fear of impending death

43. A palliative care patient receiving intrathecal combination opioid/local anesthetic administration for management of intractable neuropathic pain complains of feeling lightheaded. The palliative care nurse should:

a. Reassure the patient that this is a common adverse effect of intrathecal analgesia.
b. Prepare for imminent respiratory failure.
c. Place a Foley catheter to relieve urinary retention.
d. Check the patient's blood pressure and prepare to administer IV fluid and ephedrine if the patient is hypotensive.

44. A 41-year-old patient with advanced ovarian cancer reports feeling hopelessness and despair. All of the following are appropriate nursing interventions for helping patients maintain hope at the end of life EXCEPT:

a. Withholding bad news
b. Using humor when appropriate
c. Anticipating and treating distressing physical symptoms
d. Encouraging patients to use positive self-talk

45. All of the following are appropriate patients for palliative care team involvement EXCEPT:

a. A 59-year-old with progressive congestive heart failure refusing cardiac transplantation
b. A 47-year-old with progressive AIDS who is not requiring any analgesics
c. A 31-year-old with ALS who wants to "make the most of my limited time left"
d. A 61-year-old with chronic myelogenous leukemia that is currently in remission but likely to recur

46. A hospice patient is taking dexamethasone for treatment of cancer-related loss of appetite. Which of the following is an adverse effect of corticosteroids?

a. Gastric ulcers
b. Hypoglycemia
c. Hypotension
d. Cerebral edema

47. All of the following are features of late-stage Parkinson's disease EXCEPT:

a. Difficulty communicating
b. Inability to ambulate
c. Cognitive impairment
d. Weight gain

48. A 41-year-old leukemia patient is started on morphine and complains of nausea. Which of the following is most accurate regarding nausea and vomiting due to opioids?

a. Nausea and vomiting often improve within several days of starting opioids.
b. Nausea and vomiting only occur with oral administration of opioids.
c. Antiemetic medications are not useful for treating opioid-associated nausea and vomiting.
d. Cannabinoids (e.g., marijuana) are the first-line therapy for opioid-associated nausea.

49. A 41-year-old breast cancer patient with constipation reports episodes of stool incontinence, characterized by occasional small-volume, non-bloody liquid stools that occur without associated warning or discomfort. The most likely explanation for this is:

a. Chemotherapy-related secretory diarrhea
b. Hypercalcemia
c. Liquid stool leakage around impacted stool (i.e., overflow incontinence)
d. Acute infectious enteritis

50. Anxiety and depression are distinguished from normal, expected emotional reactions to life-threatening illness primarily by:

a. Patient's gender
b. Severity and duration of psychiatric symptoms
c. Patient's life expectancy
d. Patient's prior mental health history

51. The palliative care team is caring for a patient with advanced pancreatic cancer who has an opiate addiction. All of the following are appropriate strategies for pain management in a patient with opiate addiction EXCEPT:

a. Empower the patient in taking control of his medication regimen by providing several weeks' worth of opiate analgesics.
b. Maximize use of nonopioid and nonpharmacologic adjuvant analgesics.
c. Optimize use of sustained-release opioids rather than immediate-release opioids.
d. Consult and utilize members of the care team who have addiction expertise.

52. The husband of a hospice patient who recently died of breast cancer is concerned that his 4-year-old daughter does not accept that her mother has died because she is playful when she is at a friend's house. The nurse should explain that:

a. Normal grief in children her age includes the expression of all emotions, including joy.
b. Playing at a friend's house so soon after the death of her mother is probably confusing her.
c. The child should be evaluated for complicated grief.
d. The child's ability to play is a sign that her grieving is complete.

53. A hospice patient is receiving rectally administered morphine for pain control. Advantages of rectal opioid administration include all of the following EXCEPT:

a. More reliable and predictable opioid absorption with rectal administration than with oral administration
b. Easy administration technique for providers or family members
c. Usable in patients who have bowel obstruction or dysphagia
d. Variety of opioids and dosages available for rectal administration

54. A patient with terminal anal cancer has a marked reduction in his appetite as his disease progresses, but reports that his pain and nausea are well controlled and that he is "eating what feels right to me." The patient's wife is extremely distressed by the patient's appetite reduction and asks how she can get him to eat more. The most appropriate intervention in this case is:

a. Education and reassurance that decreased appetite is an expected change as terminal illness progresses
b. Encouraging the patient's wife to offer him larger amounts of food at each meal
c. Placement of a nasogastric tube for nutritional supplementation
d. Initiation of corticosteroid medication

55. Which of the following statements is most accurate regarding hypodermoclysis (subcutaneous fluid infusion) in the palliative care patient?

a. Hypodermoclysis catheter placement is more painful than IV catheter placement.
b. Hypodermoclysis catheters can be placed and used in the home hospice setting.
c. Hypodermoclysis can only be used for bolus administration, not continuous fluid infusion.
d. Hypodermoclysis is associated with a higher incidence of accidental air emboli.

56. A home hospice patient covered under the Medicare Hospice Benefit needs a walker and commode. The nurse should explain that:

a. The patient will need to be transferred to a nursing home to have access to that equipment.
b. Only home medical equipment delivery costs are covered under the Medicare Hospice Benefit.
c. The Medicare Hospice Benefit does not cover home medical equipment.
d. Home medical equipment delivery, training, and maintenance are covered under the Medicare Hospice Benefit.

57. A patient with multiple sclerosis and dysphagia tells the nurse that he has no interest in diet modifications (e.g., pureed) but still wants to eat. The nurse should explain that:

a. Various mechanical maneuvers can help with dysphagia.
b. It is a good time for the patient to consider non-oral nutrition.
c. Without diet modifications, it is not safe for the patient to eat orally.
d. Many patients feel the same way about diet modifications.

58. A hospice patient taking amitriptyline for the treatment of neuropathic pain develops urinary retention, tachycardia, and blurred vision. This is most likely due to which of the following adverse effects of amitriptyline?

a. Cardiac arrhythmia
b. Sexual dysfunction
c. Anticholinergic effect
d. Excessive perspiration

59. Properties of an analgesic medication to treat breakthrough pain in the hospice patient should include all of the following EXCEPT:

a. It has a rapid onset.
b. It can be administered on an as-needed (i.e., PRN) basis.
c. It is long-acting.
d. It uses the oral administration route if possible.

60. All of the following are possible complications of constipation in the palliative care patient EXCEPT:

a. Fever
b. Agitation
c. Abdominal pain
d. Urinary retention

61. The palliative care nurse is caring for a dying patient whose family members have long-standing ineffective and hostile communication techniques with one another. With regard to providing information to family members, the nurse should:

a. Communicate primarily with the most opinionated and forceful family member.
b. Communicate important information individually to family members rather than depending on open lines of communication.
c. Insist that the family pull together for the sake of the patient.
d. Have a different palliative care team member communicating with each family member.

62. The drug of choice for opioid-related nausea in the palliative care patient is:

a. Dexamethasone
b. Metoclopramide
c. Naloxone
d. Haloperidol

63. A 53-year-old patient with hepatic cancer is changing from morphine to oxycodone because of intolerable adverse effects. His pain has been well controlled on the morphine regimen. The first step in changing this patient to oxycodone is:

a. Calculate the total 24-hour dose of morphine with the current analgesic regimen.
b. Begin oxycodone at the identical morphine dose (e.g., replace 10 mg of morphine with 10 mg of oxycodone).
c. Start oxycodone at 125-150% of the calculated equianalgesic dose.
d. Start oxycodone at an equianalgesic dose while continuing the current morphine dose for 1-2 days.

64. A 19-year-old patient with terminal leukemia is not expected to survive more than 2-3 hours. The hospice nurse would expect all of the following features in this patient EXCEPT:

a. Noisy breathing secondary to pooled oral secretions
b. Decreased level of awareness and responsiveness
c. Warm, pink extremities
d. Marked decrease in urine output

65. A patient is being treated with palliative ("terminal") sedation for management of refractory, severe agitation at the end of life. The responsibilities of the nurse include all of the following EXCEPT:

a. Communicate with family members about what to expect.
b. Monitor the patient's response to sedative titration.
c. Discontinue other comfort measures as the patient becomes more sedated.
d. Use available education and support to address personal or professional concerns about palliative sedation.

66. A cancer patient reveals to the hospice nurse that he has been refusing pain medication because "I deserve to suffer for all the pain I've caused in my family." The hospice nurse should:

a. Tell the patient that he must be depressed.
b. Continue discussion with the patient to elicit more information about the patient's feelings and beliefs.
c. Tell a family member what the patient said.
d. Tell the patient that God would not want him to suffer this way.

67. A patient with terminal cancer has anorexia/cachexia syndrome (ACS). One of the features differentiating cachexia from anorexia is:

a. Cachexia is associated with loss of adipose tissue rather than lean muscle.
b. Anorexia in cancer patients is caused by a systemic inflammatory response.
c. Cachexia-associated weight loss cannot be reversed with increased nutritional intake.
d. Anorexia leads to equal loss of fat and muscle tissue.

68. The palliative care nurse is treating a patient who has delirium that is not caused by alcohol or drug withdrawal. The most appropriate medication for the nurse to administer in this case is:

a. Haloperidol
b. Phenobarbital
c. Lorazepam
d. Morphine

69. Which of the following is most accurate regarding artificial hydration in the patient with terminal illness?

a. Artificial hydration is not considered a medical intervention.
b. Artificial hydration causes emotional distress in most family members.
c. Withholding artificial hydration is inappropriate in patients with dysphagia.
d. Artificial hydration may add to patient suffering.

70. A hospice patient with hepatic cancer has little money and is receiving hospice benefits from Medicaid. He is not taking his prescribed nausea medication because it is not paid for by Medicaid. The nurse's best action is to:

a. Advise the patient to seek out private insurance coverage.
b. Help the patient get an antiemetic medication that is covered by Medicaid.
c. Advise the patient to contact Medicaid to get authorization for the medication.
d. Advise the patient to pay for the medication out-of-pocket.

71. A 27-year-old hospice patient with testicular cancer expresses feeling abandoned by God. Spiritual support by the nurse should include:

a. Active listening and acknowledgment of the patient's suffering
b. Sharing the nurse's religious beliefs with the patient
c. Reminding the patient that the nurse is not the appropriate person to offer spiritual guidance
d. Urging the patient to acknowledge ways in which his situation could be worse

72. The palliative care nurse is attempting to elicit quality-of-life priorities in a patient with life-threatening illness. Among the following, the most effective question the nurse can ask the patient is:

a. "How do you want your loved ones to commemorate you after you've died?"
b. "Have you had the experience of someone close to you dying?"
c. "How has your illness interfered with your daily life?"
d. "Would you want to be put on a ventilator if you stopped breathing?"

73. A dying patient develops noisy, congested-sounding breathing (i.e., "death rattle"), which is very distressing to the patient's loved ones. All of the following medications are appropriate for management of excessive upper respiratory tract secretions in the dying patient EXCEPT:

a. Hyoscine hydrobromide
b. Atropine sulfate
c. Albuterol
d. Glycopyrrolate

74. A 52-year-old patient with advanced prostate cancer, who requires increased morphine dosage for pain, develops involuntary movements. The hospice nurse notes that the patient is alert and responsive and is having intermittent, brief jerking movements of his arms and legs. Which of the following is the most likely explanation for these findings?

a. Superior vena cava obstruction
b. Metastatic brain disease
c. Anxiety
d. Morphine-induced myoclonus

75. When a patient confides to the nurse that he is underreporting his pain because he wants "to be strong for my wife and kids," the hospice nurse should explain that:

a. Other patients would live longer if they were all as strong as he is.
b. Accurate reporting of pain will help ensure that all of the patient's goals for palliative care are addressed.
c. Minimizing pain medication use will help prevent addiction.
d. Pain is an inevitable and universal component of end-of-life care.

76. Instructions for patients and caregivers regarding proper use of transdermal fentanyl (i.e., patch) should include all of the following EXCEPT:

a. Do not take other opioid medications while the fentanyl patch is in place.
b. Do not apply heat (e.g., hot water bottle) over the fentanyl patch.
c. Fold together the adhesive surfaces of used patches and discard in a location away from pets and children.
d. Change the patch every 72 hours.

77. A 39-year-old hospice patient with melanoma develops back pain, bilateral foot paresthesia, and urinary retention. The hospice nurse notes gait changes consistent with bilateral leg weakness. Which of the following is the most likely explanation for these findings?

a. Brain metastatic disease
b. Seizure
c. Degenerative arthritis of the vertebral column
d. Spinal metastatic disease

78. A family member asks the hospice nurse which of the senses are maintained when someone is dying. The nurse answers that the sense that is thought to be preserved longest is:

a. Sight
b. Hearing
c. Taste
d. Smell

79. A 51-year-old patient with prostate cancer has had adequate pain control with parenteral morphine and is being converted to oral morphine. He has been receiving a total of morphine 30 mg IV over 24 hours and is being converted to sustained-release oral morphine administered twice daily. The conversion rate from IV to oral morphine is 1:3. Assuming equianalgesic dosing (100% dosage conversion), which of the following is the correct oral morphine regimen for this patient?

a. Oral sustained-release morphine 90 mg twice daily
b. Oral sustained-release morphine 45 mg twice daily
c. Oral sustained-release morphine 5 mg twice daily
d. Oral sustained-release morphine 10 mg twice daily

80. A primary care physician tells the palliative care nurse that a 51-year-old terminally ill patient is not eligible for the Medicare Hospice Benefit because the patient is not willing to sign a "do not resuscitate" (DNR) order. The palliative care nurse should:

a. Urge the patient to sign a DNR order so that he will be eligible for the Medicare Hospice Benefit.
b. Encourage the physician to find out if the eligibility requirements are different in a neighboring state.
c. Inform the physician that a patient younger than 65 years of age is not eligible for the Medicare Hospice Benefit.
d. Inform the physician that a signed DNR order is not an eligibility requirement for the Medicare Hospice Benefit.

81. Which of the following is most accurate regarding the effects of dehydration in the terminally ill hospice patient?

a. Dehydration leads to increased respiratory secretions at the end of life.
b. Dehydration is associated with increased risk for pulmonary edema.
c. Dehydration is associated with increased risk for pressure injuries.
d. Dehydration is associated with decreased risk of drug accumulation.

82. All of the following are common barriers to providing optimal palliative care to the elderly population EXCEPT:

a. Difficulty assessing pain in the elderly patient with impaired communication and cognition
b. Unwillingness of the elderly population to discuss end-of-life care
c. Increased medication-related complications in elderly patients due to age-related physiological factors
d. Lack of adequate support and knowledge of palliative care in most nursing homes

83. A cancer patient asks his provider not to disclose the expected prognosis until he feels more "emotionally prepared" to hear it. The most appropriate response is to:

a. Inform the patient that not knowing the prognosis will make it difficult for him to make the most of the time he has left.
b. Disclose the prognosis to the patient's family members and ask them to convey the information to the patient.
c. Have the patient set a date for when he feels he will be ready for the information.
d. Honor the patient's request and continue ongoing psychosocial assessment and support.

84. To prevent pressure injury development, caregivers should provide full-body passive repositioning for the immobile palliative care patient approximately every:

a. 2 hours
b. 24 hours
c. 10 minutes
d. 6 hours

85. The process of "titrating to effect" regarding analgesic medications refers to:

a. Doubling analgesic dose until adequate pain relief is achieved
b. Increasing or decreasing analgesic dose based on patient's pain-relief needs and response to dosage changes
c. Increasing analgesic dose until adverse effects of pain medication develop
d. Increasing analgesic dose until patient no longer appears to be in pain

86. Common indications for corticosteroid (e.g., dexamethasone) use in palliative care patients include all of the following EXCEPT:

a. Bone pain
b. Delirium
c. Metastatic spinal cord compression
d. Anorexia (loss of appetite)

87. A 59-year-old hospice patient with terminal prostate cancer describes being in the presence of a family member who has been dead for many years. The patient does not appear agitated or uncomfortable. The hospice nurse should:

a. Administer a sedative medication to treat the patient's delirium.
b. Inform the patient that he is hallucinating.
c. Affirm the patient's experience.
d. Administer supplemental oxygen.

88. A palliative care patient develops carcinoid syndrome secondary to a metastatic carcinoid tumor. All of the following are typical features of carcinoid syndrome EXCEPT:

a. Constipation
b. Flushing
c. Abdominal cramping
d. Wheezing

89. A hospice patient being treated for severe *Clostridioides difficile* diarrhea is resistant to wearing diapers despite copious diarrhea and limited mobility. The most appropriate nursing intervention is:

a. Offer disposable underpads and a bedside commode in place of diapers.
b. Avoid barrier ointments to the perirectal area.
c. Advise decreased oral fluid intake.
d. Tell the patient that diapers are his best choice for hygiene.

90. A patient with prostate cancer complains of a heavy sensation in both legs and back pain, which is exacerbated by lying flat and coughing. The palliative care nurse should suspect which of the following conditions in this patient?

a. Spinal cord compression
b. Myoclonus
c. Seizure
d. Overexertion

91. A patient with terminal breast cancer is experiencing agitation, sleep disturbance, and intermittent confusion, consistent with delirium. Supportive interventions should include all of the following EXCEPT:

a. Maintain familiar sounds and smells in the patient's environment.
b. Cover windows to decrease the patient's day/night awareness.
c. Avoid excessive auditory and visual stimuli.
d. Offer gentle reassurance, repeated as needed.

92. After the death of a hospice patient at home, the patient's remaining opiate analgesic medications should be:

a. Dealt with at the family's discretion
b. Kept in the home out of the reach of children
c. Returned to the hospice agency for use with other patients
d. Disposed of according to federal and hospice agency guidelines

93. A 31-year-old hospice patient with end-stage AIDS tells the nurse, "I'm going to die before I really had a chance to do anything." The nurse's best intervention is:

a. Remind the patient that many people die at a much younger age than he will.
b. Encourage the patient to share memories of life events, relationships, and conflicts.
c. Advise the patient to make medical decisions that will maximize his survival time.
d. Tell the patient, "I can understand how you must feel."

94. The palliative care nurse is discussing the benefits versus burdens of initiating noninvasive positive pressure ventilation (BiPAP) in a terminally ill patient with dyspnea. All of the following should be included in this discussion EXCEPT:

a. How the benefits and burdens of BiPAP specifically apply to the patient's end-of-life goals
b. Potential complications of BiPAP use
c. Potential impact of BiPAP use on the patient's symptoms
d. Education that the decision to initiate BiPAP is irreversible

95. A palliative care patient taking anticholinergic medication for treatment of urinary incontinence will most likely report which of the following adverse effects?

a. Blurry vision
b. Dry mouth
c. Chest pain
d. Diarrhea

96. Supportive measures for enhancing comfort in the palliative care patient with fever include all of the following EXCEPT:

a. Antipyretic medication
b. Dry clothes and linens
c. Mouth care
d. Cooling blankets

97. All of the following conditions may increase the likelihood of adverse effects due to nonsteroidal anti-inflammatory medications (e.g., ibuprofen) EXCEPT:

a. Renal dysfunction
b. Gastrointestinal bleeding
c. Platelet dysfunction
d. Pancreatic insufficiency

98. A terminally ill hospice patient with ovarian cancer becomes bedbound and less responsive as a result of disease progression. The most appropriate approach to managing the development of pressure injuries in this patient is:

a. Treatment of wound pain to maintain patient comfort
b. Frequent debridement and wound cleaning
c. Daily wet-to-dry dressing changes
d. Obtain wound culture to guide antibiotic treatment

99. A 57-year-old man with liver cirrhosis due to long-term alcohol abuse develops confusion and decreased level of consciousness, consistent with hepatic encephalopathy. Which of the following lab findings would most likely explain this patient's symptoms?

a. Elevated serum ammonia
b. Elevated serum alanine aminotransferase (ALT)
c. Elevated serum white blood cell count
d. Elevated prothrombin time (PT)

100. A patient with breast cancer has progressive upper-extremity swelling due to lymphedema. The mainstay of treatment for extremity lymphedema is:

a. Diuretics
b. Exercise
c. External compression
d. Diet

101. Stool impaction commonly leads to all of the following urinary tract complications EXCEPT:

a. Urinary incontinence
b. Urinary retention
c. Urinary tract infection
d. Hematuria

102. Appropriate nursing intervention for assisting patients and families in preparing for death includes all of the following EXCEPT:

a. Teaching the patient and family members about the dying process
b. Assisting patients and families with funeral arrangements
c. Helping patients identify and accomplish things they'd like to do before they die
d. Advising family to take the patient to the nearest hospital for death pronouncement

103. Which of the following factors is associated with increased risk of elder abuse at the end of life?

a. Low socioeconomic status of patient
b. Non-family caregiver
c. Caregiver with active substance abuse
d. Female patient

104. A patient with oral cancer covered under the Medicare Hospice Benefit is due for the 180-day hospice recertification so that coverage can continue. All of the following are required components of the 180-day hospice recertification EXCEPT:

a. Physician certification that the patient's life expectancy is 6 months or less based on expected disease course
b. Brief summary of clinical information supporting the assertion that life expectancy is 6 months or less
c. Physician certification that the patient has a confirmed malignancy
d. Documentation of a face-to-face visit in which clinical information supporting the patient's hospice eligibility was gathered

105. The most accurate statement about the benefit of interdisciplinary collaboration as it relates to palliative care is:

a. Interdisciplinary collaboration utilizes joint decision-making and responsibility to meet a common goal.
b. Interdisciplinary collaboration expedites care by relegating treatment decisions to one provider.
c. Interdisciplinary collaboration in palliative care results in increased Medicare reimbursement.
d. Interdisciplinary collaboration decreases the responsibility and accountability of each individual team member.

106. Physical assessment of the patient with xerostomia may reveal all of the following EXCEPT:

a. Halitosis
b. Thick, sticky saliva
c. Oral ulcerations
d. Salivary pooling

107. Bisphosphonates (e.g., pamidronate) are used in palliative care patients for treatment of both hypercalcemia and:

a. Neuropathic pain
b. Dyspnea
c. Bone pain
d. Urinary retention

108. A 48-year-old patient has terminal lung cancer that requires large doses of oral opioids for pain control. The patient complains of abdominal bloating and hard, infrequent stools that require straining to pass. Nonpharmacologic measures for treatment of opioid-related constipation include all of the following EXCEPT:

a. Increased oral fluid intake
b. Decreased physical activity
c. Increased dietary fiber intake
d. Sitting upright during defecation

109. A hospice patient being cared for at home develops seizures. The patient does not have IV access and is unable to take oral medication. The most appropriate initial pharmacologic intervention for acute seizure management in this patient is:

a. Intramuscular dexamethasone
b. Subcutaneous phenobarbital
c. Rectal diazepam
d. Intramuscular fosphenytoin

110. The primary risk factor for the development of pressure injuries is:

a. Advanced age
b. Skin moisture
c. Low socioeconomic status
d. Immobility

111. The widow of a hospice patient who died two months ago reports frequent crying, poor concentration, difficulty sleeping, and feelings of disbelief that her husband is "gone." This is most consistent with:

a. Anxiety disorder
b. Complicated grief
c. A major depressive episode
d. Uncomplicated grief

112. The partner of a patient with metastatic colorectal cancer asks the hospice nurse to tell her when the patient is "close to death" so that she can call other family members to come to the bedside before the patient dies. The nurse's most appropriate response is:

a. "There is no way to tell that a patient is close to death."
b. "I can teach you to recognize the signs indicating that your partner is likely close to death."
c. "It would probably be best if your partner dies in an inpatient hospice facility."
d. "Most patients prefer not to burden their family members with being present at the time of death."

113. A 61-year-old hospice patient is pain-free on his current opioid regimen but is experiencing persistent, intolerable sedation. All of the following are reasonable therapeutic strategies in this patient EXCEPT:

a. Trial of reduced opioid dosage
b. Trial of alternate opioid medication
c. Addition of prokinetic gastrointestinal agent (e.g., metoclopramide)
d. Addition of psychostimulant medication (e.g., methylphenidate)

114. A 44-year-old patient with breast cancer complains of shortness of breath, abdominal pressure, and nausea due to malignant ascites. The intervention most likely to provide immediate relief in this patient is:

a. Oral diuretics
b. Paracentesis
c. Oral sodium restriction
d. IV fluid administration

115. A 61-year-old patient with terminal prostate cancer and an indwelling urinary catheter complains of severe, intermittent cramping pain in the suprapubic region. All of the following etiologies would explain the patient's symptoms EXCEPT:

a. Urinary tract infection
b. Urinary catheter occlusion
c. Excess oral fluid intake
d. History of pelvic radiation therapy

116. An adult patient with cystic fibrosis, who clearly articulated her preferences for end-of-life comfort care, is dying at home. As signs of impending death develop, the patient's family tells the hospice nurse that they are not ready for her to die and now "want everything done." The most appropriate response is:

a. Begin resuscitation and call 911 for transport to the nearest hospital.
b. Tell the family that it is too late to change the plan of care.
c. Gently remind the family of the patient's wishes for end-of-life care and the ultimate futility of life-extending resuscitation.
d. Tell the family that the presence of hospice team members is no longer appropriate if they change the plan of care.

117. All of the following are consistent with appropriate palliative care public policy advocacy by the palliative care nurse EXCEPT:

a. Evaluate public policy proposals related to palliative care.
b. Coordinate efforts with other professional groups to advocate for palliative care legislation.
c. Lobby policy makers on palliative care legislation to advance the nurse's personal interests.
d. Contact the media to increase public awareness of palliative care public policy issues.

118. A 51-year-old patient with terminal lung cancer wants to attend his son's college graduation (a two-hour drive) before he dies. The palliative care nurse's best response is:

a. "We'll see how you're doing on the day of his graduation."
b. "Most people aren't up to a trip like that at this stage of lung cancer."
c. "It would be better to conserve your energy so that you can have more time with your son before you die."
d. "I can help you and the rest of the care team figure out what we need to do so that you can go to your son's graduation."

119. A 61-year-old hospice patient with chronic obstructive pulmonary disease (COPD) is experiencing increased shortness of breath. The hospice nurse should teach family caregivers all of the following strategies for management of dyspnea EXCEPT:

a. Patient breathing techniques (e.g., pursed-lip breathing)
b. Giving the patient some alone time when the patient is short of breath
c. Placement of patient near an open window or fan
d. Practical strategies for maximizing the effectiveness of the patient's bronchodilator medication

120. Reflex urinary incontinence due to spinal cord compression is most effectively managed with:

a. Catheterization
b. Pelvic floor muscle training
c. Antibiotics
d. Fluid restriction

121. Assuming all of the following patients are receiving opioid medication, naloxone administration is most appropriate in which of the following clinical situations?

a. An ovarian cancer patient with irregular respirations in association with impending death
b. An unresponsive colorectal cancer patient with respiratory rate of 6 breaths/minute and oxygen saturation 84%
c. A glioblastoma patient with opioid-related constipation
d. An arousable melanoma patient with respiratory rate of 8 breaths/minute and oxygen saturation 92%

122. A patient with pancreatic cancer is experiencing neuropathic pain that is not opioid-responsive. The most appropriate clinical intervention in this patient is:

a. Increased frequency of opioid administration
b. Trial of bisphosphonate medication
c. Palliative ("terminal") sedation
d. Trial of tricyclic antidepressant medication

123. A 24-year-old hospice patient with lymphoma is complaining of chest pain. A physiological pain assessment should include all of the following EXCEPT:

a. Intensity of pain
b. Quality of pain
c. Contributory emotional stressors
d. Aggravating/alleviating factors

124. A 47-year-old bedbound hospice patient with terminal ovarian cancer has gradually reduced food and fluid intake over the course of several weeks and ultimately stops eating and drinking altogether. The most likely explanation for this is:

a. Malignant bowel obstruction
b. Impending death
c. Depression
d. Inadequate pain control

125. The palliative care nurse is caring for a 49-year-old patient with bone pain due to metastatic breast cancer. The nurse notes that this patient complains of more severe pain than patients the nurse has cared for in the past who had similar metastatic bone disease. The most likely explanation for this discrepancy is:

a. The patient has an undisclosed drug addiction.
b. The patient is reporting psychological pain as physical pain.
c. The patient is over-reporting physical pain as an attention-seeking behavior.
d. The patient's pain is a reflection of the multidimensional factors unique to this patient.

126. Among the following, the most appropriate analgesic medication for initial treatment of mild pain in the palliative care patient is:

a. Morphine
b. Dexamethasone
c. Acetaminophen
d. Codeine

127. The family of Jack, a 41-year-old patient with AIDS, tells the hospice nurse that they are canceling their annual New Year's Eve movie night because they don't want the patient to feel bad if he is too ill to attend. The nurse's best response is:

a. "It's great that you're taking Jack's feelings into account and canceling movie night."
b. "Jack will feel even worse if he knows you canceled movie night on his account."
c. "Let's try to figure out a way for Jack to get the care he needs without canceling an important family event."
d. "You can always have the movie night after Jack dies."

128. When a provider is breaking bad news to a patient, all of the following are barriers to effective communication EXCEPT:

a. Multiple family members are present.
b. The provider uses complex medical terms.
c. The language spoken by the patient is different than that of the provider.
d. The provider discloses incomplete information because of the belief that the news is "too much to handle."

129. A 51-year-old patient with COPD who has not had any prior involvement with palliative care is being discharged from the hospital and enrolling in home hospice care. The role of the palliative care nurse in this process may include all of the following EXCEPT:

a. Participate in formulating a plan of care for the transition to home hospice care.
b. Certify that the patient has an anticipated life expectancy of 6 months or less.
c. Assist in coordinating home delivery of medications and supplies that the patient requires.
d. Teach the patient and family members how to administer oxygen at home.

130. All of the following are important factors in maintaining the psychosocial well-being of palliative care nurses EXCEPT:

a. Teaching nurses how to identify signs of stress and burnout in themselves and colleagues
b. Teaching nurses the importance of making time for self-care
c. Teaching nurses to put their patients' needs before their own
d. Encouraging supportive and caring relationships among nurse colleagues

131. Family members of a hospice patient are recommending that the patient try massage therapy for the treatment of cancer pain that is currently well-controlled with opioids. When asked for his or her opinion, the hospice nurse should respond that:

a. "Many patients find massage therapy a helpful additional therapy for treating cancer pain."
b. "Alternative medicine is not a proven science."
c. "Massage usually doesn't help with pain due to advanced cancer."
d. "Massage therapy could make your pain medications less effective."

132. A palliative care patient with metastatic lung cancer tells the nurse that his opioid pain medication is no longer adequately controlling his pain. Which of the following signs would be most consistent with psychological dependence (i.e., addiction) to opioids?

a. Physical symptoms of withdrawal when opioid is discontinued
b. Need for increased dose after long-term use of opioid medication
c. Requesting medication before the prescribed dose interval
d. Compulsive opioid use despite negative effects

133. A 69-year-old patient with renal cell carcinoma consistently reports severe back pain 1 hour before scheduled pain medication is due. This is most consistent with:

a. Incident pain
b. Spontaneous pain
c. End-of-dose failure
d. Drug-seeking behavior

134. An ethics conference is arranged to discuss conflict between a hospice patient, family members, and medical providers regarding withdrawal of artificial hydration. The most appropriate participation of the patient's primary hospice nurse in this conference consists of:

a. Observation without active participation
b. Active participation and advocacy for a patient-centered care plan
c. Providing relevant information about nursing tasks associated with the plan of care
d. No direct involvement

135. All of the following diseases are characterized by irreversible, progressive neurological decline EXCEPT:

a. Huntington's disease
b. Multiple sclerosis
c. Alzheimer's disease
d. Amyotrophic lateral sclerosis

136. The National Consensus Project maintains the Clinical Practice Guidelines for Quality Palliative Care, which establish clinical practice guidelines for:

a. Palliative care provision across all age groups and practice settings
b. Inpatient hospice programs
c. Adult patients with life-threatening conditions
d. Federally funded palliative care programs

137. In the palliative care patient with end-stage congestive heart failure, opioid medication use would be most helpful for treating:

a. Chest pain
b. Constipation
c. Fatigue
d. Edema

138. The American Nurses Association's position on appropriate nursing care for pain management at the end of life is best summarized as:

a. Opioid analgesics should be titrated to effect up to the maximum established medication dosage as determined by professional standards.
b. Administration of placebo (in place of analgesic medication) is justified if there is nursing concern for respiratory depression.
c. Increased analgesic dosing for treatment of pain is justified if there is no chance of hastening death.
d. Analgesic medication should be administered in the dosage required to achieve adequate pain control.

139. The most common presenting symptom of metastatic disease in the bone is:

a. Numbness
b. Pain
c. Weakness
d. Hypercalcemia

140. Palliative care nurses are in the best position to provide compassionate patient care when the primary educational and professional emphasis is on:

a. Maintaining professional roles
b. Developing an authentic caring relationship with the patients
c. Providing maximally efficient care
d. Employing the most up-to-date technological palliative care advances

141. A 71-year-old woman with progressive COPD has a prolonged coughing episode during dinner. The following day, she develops fever, increased respiratory distress, and worsening oxygenation. This is most consistent with:

a. Pulmonary embolism
b. Myocardial infarction
c. Aspiration pneumonia
d. Pneumothorax

142. Which of the following statements is most accurate about the provision of hospice care in nursing homes under the Medicare Hospice Benefit?

a. The hospice patient in a nursing home receives the same hospice care services that he or she would receive at home.
b. Hospice care is significantly overused in nursing home patients.
c. The Medicare Hospice Benefit does not cover hospice care in the nursing home setting.
d. Hospice care in the nursing home setting is provided exclusively by the nursing home staff.

143. With regard to elderly patients, which of the following statements about falls is most accurate?

a. Mortality rates are similar pre-fall and post-fall.
b. It is difficult to predict which elderly patients are at increased risk for falls.
c. Falls are uncommon in elderly patients who reside in nursing homes.
d. Underlying medical conditions are a frequent contributing cause of falls in the elderly population.

144. A team consisting of a physician, a nurse, a social worker, a psychologist, the patient's family, and the patient, makes up the interdisciplinary palliative care team for a terminally ill patient. To provide optimal palliative care for the patient, the most effective model for collaboration among the team members is:

a. Individual members of the care team independently providing recommendations to the patient in their area of expertise
b. Physician coordination of other team members' recommendations before presenting a plan of care to the patient
c. Regular meetings with all team members collaborating on a unified plan of care
d. A meeting of palliative care team involvement at the onset to formulate a plan of care that will be in place until the patient's death

145. A patient in a hospital-based palliative care program wants to transfer to home hospice care. The best way to facilitate transfer for this patient is:

a. Give the patient a list of home hospice agencies that provide care near his or her home.
b. Establish direct communication with the patient's home hospice provider to ensure smooth transfer of care.
c. Give the patient a copy of his or her latest care plan to provide to home hospice providers.
d. Ask the patient to provide home hospice agency contact information so that hospital records can be sent.

146. The nurse most likely to enjoy long-term satisfaction in palliative care nursing views his or her job primarily as:

a. An opportunity to alleviate patient suffering through a meaningful patient-nurse relationship
b. An opportunity to master the tasks of palliative nursing
c. A source of career advancement opportunity
d. A way to earn a living

147. The hospice nurse asks a 69-year-old patient with multiple myeloma why he doesn't participate in interdisciplinary team discussions about his plan of care. He replies, "I don't know as much about this disease as all of you." The nurse's best response is:

a. "Your participation will help us make the best plan of care because you know more than any of us about your goals and preferences."
b. "You need to be more assertive during team meetings."
c. "Whoever you've chosen as your healthcare power of attorney can come to the meetings instead."
d. "You don't have to go to the meetings if they make you uncomfortable."

148. All of the following are within the scope of practice for the hospice home health aide EXCEPT:

a. Educating family care providers about skin and mouth care
b. Performing light housekeeping tasks (e.g., meal preparation, laundry)
c. Educating family care providers about the use of a vascular catheter
d. Transferring patient from bed to chair

149. Assessment of the impact of affective/psychological factors on a palliative care patient's pain will focus on the:

a. Location of pain
b. Patient's emotional responses to pain
c. Patient's cultural beliefs about pain
d. Type of pain (e.g., neuropathic)

150. A 45-year-old patient with breast cancer develops skin itching, redness, and flaking of the chest wall after radiation therapy. Which of the following is most accurate regarding dermatologic adverse effects of radiation therapy?

a. Radiation-associated skin changes are rare unless the patient is being treated for a primary skin cancer.
b. Radiation-associated skin changes typically appear 2-3 weeks after initiation of treatment.
c. Tight-fitting clothing around the treatment area is helpful for managing radiation-associated skin changes.
d. Topical steroids are contraindicated for treatment of radiation-associated skin reactions.

Answers and Explanations

1. C: Hyperkalemia (elevated serum potassium level) is a common complication of end-stage renal failure as a result of diminished ability of the failing kidney to excrete potassium. Life-threatening hyperkalemia is often asymptomatic until sudden cardiac arrest occurs. Chronic renal failure is associated with several metabolic abnormalities. These include anemia, hypocalcemia, hyperphosphatemia, metabolic acidosis, and hypoalbuminemia. Sudden cardiac death in the patient with renal failure is most likely due to elevated serum potassium levels.

2. A: In addition to the serious psychological harm caused by uncontrolled pain in the palliative care patient, there are several harmful physiological effects of inadequate treatment of pain. Increased heart rate and blood pressure lead to increased metabolic demand and increased myocardial stress. Decreased mobility due to inadequate pain relief increases the patient's risk of pressure injuries, muscle wasting, and deep venous thrombosis. Gastric motility generally slows, leading to ileus. Risk of atelectasis and pneumonia are increased in patients who are breathing shallowly because of uncontrolled pain in the chest or chest wall. Excessive sedative effects of pain medications may impair the patient's ability to interact with loved ones, but this should be managed with medication adjustments or use of psychoactive stimulants. Uncontrolled pain does not enhance a patient's ability to have meaningful interactions with anyone. Finally, adequate pain control should not interfere with management of the patient's primary disease.

3. A: Supporting the patient in decision-making with regard to advanced care planning is an extremely important component of palliative care nursing. Advanced care planning should, ideally, begin before the late stages of a terminal illness; it is difficult for patients and loved ones to consider advanced care planning in the setting of an acute decompensation. Advanced care planning should occur over the course of several conversations to allow patients time to reflect and process what are, for most patients, emotionally challenging issues. Planning should address the patient's goals regarding life-sustaining therapy (e.g., code status), preparation for the possibility of the patient becoming incapable of decision-making, and a designated proxy for decision-making if the patient is unable to do so. It usually provides a great deal of relief to both patients and loved ones when end-of-life decisions are made ahead of time in keeping with the patient's values and goals.

4. C: The application of heat to an area of pain results in multiple physiological effects. Blood flow, tissue compliance, and muscle fiber relaxation increase in response to the application of a heat source. Heat also results in decreased nerve transmission of pain signals to the brain and spinal cord (via effects on both temperature and pressure receptors), which in turn enhances muscle relaxation and blood flow. Heat may be applied in a variety of ways, most of which are easy to use for both care providers and patients. Options include submersion (of either part of the body or the whole patient) in warm water, radiant heaters, hot packs, heating pads, hot water bottles, and heat wraps. Heat should not usually be applied over areas of decreased sensation because of the risk of burns.

5. B: The Medicare Hospice Benefit provides for four different levels of hospice care, depending on the needs of the terminally ill patient. Routine home care (most common) is provided in the patient's home or a long-term care facility. Inpatient respite care consists of up to 5 consecutive days of inpatient hospice care to provide relief to a family caregiver. General inpatient hospice care is provided for the patient whose home environment is no longer a safe care setting or the patient whose symptoms are no longer manageable in the home setting. Under the Medicare Hospice

Benefit, continuous home care is provided only for a crisis (psychosocial or medical) that would otherwise lead to a need for inpatient hospice care. The patient must be requiring at least 8 hours of nursing-level hospice care for it to be classified as continuous home care. Less than 8 hours of nursing-level care is classified as routine home care under the Medicare Hospice Benefit.

6. A: The nature of palliative care often leads to deep personal connections between patients, families, and the nurses taking care of them. This is one of the sources of great satisfaction and meaning for many palliative care nurses. It is common—and within the realm of palliative care nursing—to grieve when a patient dies (as long as the nurse's expressions of grief do not in any way harm the patient or family) and to keep in touch with the loved ones of past patients. It is also appropriate for the palliative care nurse to help the patient's loved ones to express their feelings and thoughts as death approaches, including goodbyes. However, if the meaningful connection that the nurse establishes with patients and families leads to the misperception that only that nurse can take good care of the patient, or if the nurse is neglecting his or her personal health or relationships, that is a good indication that professional boundaries have been crossed.

7. D: Medical care providers are often hesitant to broach the topic of a palliative care or hospice team consultation with patients and families because of their own feelings that they have somehow "failed" the patient and concern that the patient will feel like the medical providers are "giving up on them." The provider communicating with the patient should discuss the issue just as they would discuss any other subspecialty consult; emphasize the value that the experience and expertise of the palliative care team will add to the patient's care. It is important for the primary provider to emphasize that they will continue to be involved in the patient's care. This helps minimize the risk of the patient feeling abandoned. Discussing palliative or hospice care with the patient should never be used as the means of disclosing that there are no further curative therapeutic options for the patient's disease. That conversation should be conducted in a straightforward and compassionate way before broaching the topic of hospice care.

8. B: Caregiver education is an important component of palliative care nursing. Depending on the specifics of the patient's illness and care setting, caregivers may need to become familiar and comfortable with medication administration, wound care, patient transfer and positioning, and use of equipment, such as urinary or vascular catheters, oxygen delivery devices, and colostomy bags. Family care providers should be given ample time and opportunities to learn these new skills in the way that works best for them. This may include reading written materials, watching demonstrations of proper technique, or practicing skills with the nurse present for guidance and correction. Although in some cases it will be most appropriate for other care providers to perform a certain task, family members who are taught these skills in a compassionate, patient, and empowering way can usually perform them competently and comfortably.

9. A: Anemia is common in the palliative care patient, and etiologies include chronic disease, malignancy, chemotherapy, nutritional deficiency, renal disease, bone marrow failure, and medications. The patient with symptomatic anemia may complain of fatigue, decreased exercise tolerance, dyspnea, lightheadedness, syncope, and chest pain. Physical assessment may reveal pallor, tachycardia, hypotension, tachypnea, and cardiac murmur. Nosebleeds are increased in the patient with low platelet counts (i.e., thrombocytopenia).

10. B: Dyspnea is a subjective sensation of difficulty breathing and is very distressing for patients. Opioids are the pharmacologic therapy of choice for dyspnea in the palliative care patient. Adjunctive medications that may be helpful depending on the clinical situation include bronchodilators, diuretics, anxiolytics, and steroids. Nonpharmacologic strategies for managing dyspnea include breathing and relaxation techniques, upright positioning, sitting near an open window or fan, and supportive caregiver presence.

11. A: Hypercalcemia is associated with several cancers, most commonly breast, lung, lymphoma, and multiple myeloma. Hypercalcemia in the setting of advanced cancer may be caused by release of calcium due to bone metastases, solid tumor release of PTHrP (parathyroid hormone–related protein), or tumor production of calcitriol leading to increased intestinal calcium resorption. Hypercalcemia in cancer patients is indicative of widespread disease and is associated with a poor prognosis for long-term survival. Symptoms of elevated serum calcium levels include weakness, fatigue, nausea, and mental status changes. If treating hypercalcemia is in keeping with the patient's palliative care goals, serum calcium levels may be lowered with hydration, bisphosphonates, and calcitonin.

12. D: Tumor edema is a common complication of primary or metastatic brain tumors and may cause significant symptoms of elevated intracranial pressure, such as headache, altered mental status, and seizures. Tumor edema may be secondary to tumor cell death or tumor growth, or related to treatment (e.g., postoperative edema). The mainstay of therapy for brain tumor edema is systemic corticosteroids, most commonly dexamethasone. Mannitol may be indicated for emergent use in the patient with impending brain herniation due to cerebral edema, but is not the first-line treatment for tumor-associated brain edema. Although many patients with brain tumors require anticonvulsants to decrease risk of seizures, anticonvulsant medications do not directly treat tumor edema.

13. A: The palliative care patient with limitations in communicative ability or cognition poses a challenge to care providers when it comes to accurate and comprehensive pain assessment. Although it is far more difficult for these patients to reliably communicate the presence or source of pain, they are just as likely to experience pain as other palliative care patients. Multiple pain assessment scales exist for clinical use in cognitively impaired patients, and these may be particularly helpful when used to observe a trend in apparent pain behaviors. Nonverbal cues of discomfort, such as facial expressions, verbalizations, body language, and alterations in usual routine behaviors, are the primary source of information for pain assessment in these patients. Family members are an important resource for pain assessment in patients with limited ability to communicate.

14. D: Palliative sedation refers to the administration of sedatives (usually as a continuous infusion) in the patient with advanced, terminal disease for the treatment of severe, intractable symptoms that persist despite maximal standard therapy. The express intent of palliative sedation is to relieve patient suffering, not to hasten death. Palliative sedation is not appropriate in patients who are still pursuing curative therapies for their disease, in patients who are experiencing unpleasant symptoms or adverse effects that can be managed with other treatment strategies, or in patients who are requesting provider-assisted death.

15. D: Hiccups are involuntary contractions of the diaphragm that lead to rapid closure of the vocal cords. A wide variety of conditions may lead to persistent hiccups, including any condition that leads to irritation or compression of the diaphragm, phrenic nerve, vagus nerve, or brainstem reflex center. Persistent hiccups can be exhausting and painful, and can interfere with sleep and oral intake in the palliative care patient. Nonpharmacologic management of hiccups includes respiratory maneuvers (e.g., breath holding), pharyngeal stimulation (e.g., eating sugar, palate massage), distraction, acupuncture, and vagal nerve stimulation maneuvers. Pharmacologic agents that may be effective include muscle relaxants (e.g., baclofen), anticonvulsants, calcium channel blockers (e.g., nifedipine), antipsychotics (e.g., chlorpromazine), and agents aimed at reducing gastric distention (e.g., anti-gas medication, metoclopramide).

16. D: Massive hemorrhage is a relatively rare cause of death in the palliative care patient, but it is usually very distressing for family members (and sometimes for the patient as well). Comfort measures for the patient experiencing a massive hemorrhage include maintaining a calm and reassuring presence, covering blood (with dark towels or blankets if possible), keeping the mouth and face as clear as possible to minimize respiratory distress, and providing warm blankets for the cold sensation that typically accompanies hemorrhagic shock. If there is time and available access, opioids and/or benzodiazepines may be administered for patient discomfort or distress.

17. B: Anger is an expected and normal reaction to life-threatening illness, but it requires a compassionate, open-hearted, and mature response from the palliative care provider. It is important to name, acknowledge, validate, and inquire further about the patient's anger without getting defensive, avoidant, or condescending. Engaging the patient without taking the patient's feelings personally or treating anger as an unwelcome emotion is therapeutic, and it can help the patient explore and address the anger in an adaptive and healthy way. If a patient is physically aggressive or poses an imminent physical threat, the provider should take any necessary steps to maintain the physical safety of all involved before further engaging the patient.

18. C: Assessment of the home environment for safety risks is an important component of palliative care provision in the home setting. As the patient's condition changes, safety risks may change as well, requiring ongoing repeated assessments and interventions. For example, progressive neuromuscular disease may lead to more potential for falls, requiring support bars or removal of tripping hazards. Although it may ultimately be appropriate to change the setting of care for a patient being cared for at home, initial interventions should be geared toward increasing the safety of the home environment and reevaluating the needs of the patient and caregivers so that appropriate support can be provided.

19. B: Cultural and/or language barriers can present significant challenges in the palliative care setting. The proper use of medical interpreters can make a big difference in bridging a cultural gap between provider and patient. Interpreters should be used as far more than simple translators who repeat conversations verbatim. An interpreter can be very helpful in teaching providers about important cultural beliefs or norms as they relate to the patient's illness and plan of care. When using a language interpreter, avoid long, drawn-out statements laden with medical jargon to ensure accurate communication. The provider should address the patient when communicating via an interpreter; ideally, the provider is facing the patient, and the interpreter is to the side, where he or she can see both the provider and the patient.

20. B: Dysphagia is characterized by difficulty swallowing solids and/or liquids and may arise from a variety of underlying conditions, including cognitive impairment, weakness, mechanical obstruction, and incoordination. Presenting symptoms may include prolonged meal times, avoidance of certain foods or liquids, new movements of the head or body during meals, voice changes with eating, coughing, choking, or unexplained weight loss. Dysphagia places the patient at increased risk for aspiration and malnutrition.

21. D: Multiple factors increase the risk of suicide in the terminally ill patient, including depression, hopelessness, progressive disease, poorly controlled physical symptoms, inadequate support systems, and a history of psychiatric illness and/or substance abuse. While it is important for providers to be aware of their state laws regarding physician-assisted suicide in the terminally ill patient, the existence of such laws does not replace a full evaluation of the suicidal patient with a life-threatening illness. The provider should assess the patient's mental status, suicidal plans and their potential lethality, support systems, and any physical symptoms causing the patient distress.

22. A: Effective titration of opioid analgesics depends on multiple factors, including frequent pain assessments, clear medication orders that take into account the pharmacokinetics of the analgesic used, and a clear provider understanding of safe and effective opioid titration. Patients regularly requiring several bolus doses on top of the continuous infusion rate will benefit from an increase in basal rate to achieve better pain control. The most effective opioid titration orders will take into account the percentage dosage increase; for example, titrations of 1 mg/hr have vastly different effects depending on the starting dose. An increase from 2 mg/hr to 3 mg/hr represents a 50% increase in dosage, while an increase from 10 mg/hr to 11 mg/hr represents just a 10% increase. Moderate to severe pain will usually require a 50-100% dosage increase, while mild to moderate pain will usually respond to a 25-50% dosage increase. As always, individual patient response is the most important factor in pain medication titration.

23. B: Constipation should be anticipated and proactively treated whenever possible in the palliative care patient. This involves regular assessments of the patient's bowel habits and symptoms (e.g., bloating, abdominal pain, rectal pain) and monitoring for factors that predispose the patient to developing constipation (e.g., opioid therapy, decreased mobility, decreased oral intake). Because constipation is a virtually universal adverse effect of opioid therapy, a bowel regimen should be started concurrently with the initiation of opioid analgesics. Rectally administered therapy (e.g., enema, suppository) should be used as sparingly as possible. Manual disimpaction is indicated only if the patient is impacted and should be preceded by adequate analgesic and/or sedative medications. Osmotic laxatives should be taken with plenty of oral fluids, which may limit their use in palliative care patients.

24. C: Depression and anxiety disorders likely remain under-recognized in the terminally ill patient. Almost all patients experience sadness, sleep disturbance, and worry sometime in the course of terminal illness. In the absence of psychosis or severe psychological impairment, it is primarily the severity and duration of anxiety and depressive symptoms that determine whether a patient needs further evaluation and treatment. Some argue that the overlap between the physical symptoms of depression (weight loss, sleep disturbance, fatigue) and serious chronic illness make those symptoms unhelpful when it comes to screening. Several straightforward tools exist for anxiety and depression screening in the patient with life-threatening illness.

25. C: With the progression of life-threatening illness comes significant change as patients are forced to face declines in physical health and the ability to care for themselves. It is common for patients to feel as though they are burdening family caregivers. The hospice nurse can use a variety of strategies to help patients and families with this sense of burdening. Patients can be encouraged to openly discuss their fears and concerns about burdening loved ones; this allows providers to provide psychosocial support to the patient and to identify support services that may be helpful in alleviating patient and caregiver stress. The nurse can remind the patient that genuine expressions of appreciation for the care that loved ones provide are usually very welcome and can decrease caregivers' sense of burden. It can be helpful for the nurse to remind patients how important it is for caregivers to have a break, and to encourage use of other help (e.g., other home hospice staff). This is often very difficult for loved ones to express directly to the patient.

26. A: The hospice nurse will encounter a wide variety of family structures, dynamics, and coping styles in his or her career. What works well for one family in dealing with the serious illness and death of a loved one may not be helpful for another family. Assessment of the patient's family care providers, and assistance with the inevitable caregiver stress that accompanies end-of-life care, are important skills for the hospice nurse. Attitudes indicating that caregivers may need more evaluation or intervention include fault-finding, prolonged feelings of powerlessness, reluctance to receive suggestions or support, refusal to allow other family members to be involved in the patient's care, rigid adherence to their way of doing things, and exclusively negative expressions of feelings (e.g., anger, frustration).

27. C: Cystic fibrosis is an inherited autosomal recessive disease in which abnormally thick mucus affects the reproductive, gastrointestinal, and respiratory tracts. Cystic fibrosis causes respiratory disease, characterized by chronic infection, obstructive airway disease, and progressive decline in lung function. Death is most commonly the result of respiratory failure. The life expectancy of patients with cystic fibrosis has increased to the mid-30s as a result of advances in treatment. Adult palliative care providers will be caring for more patients with cystic fibrosis as the life expectancy of these patients continues to increase.

28. A: The essence of palliative care is providing end-of-life care that minimizes physical and spiritual pain and suffering in a manner that is consistent with the patient's specific goals and preferences. If the patient's care plan does not include specific interventions in response to vital sign abnormalities, or when the measurement of vital signs interferes with the patient's comfort, routine vital sign monitoring should be discontinued. In some cases, vital sign monitoring will be a component of the palliative care patient's plan of care. For example, if a patient with end-stage heart failure experiences chest pain when the heart rate is elevated, it may be clinically appropriate to monitor pulse with the goal of making the patient more comfortable.

29. B: Effective treatment of pain in the palliative care patient depends partly on accurate assessment of pain type, because some therapies may be more helpful than others for certain types of pain. Neuropathic pain is caused by nerve infiltration or injury and is usually described as burning, shooting, tingling, or shock-like. Somatic pain is caused by stimulation of skin, muscle, or bone, is well-localized, and is described as achy, throbbing, or dull. Visceral pain is caused by stimulation of abdominal or thoracic organs, is poorly localized, and is described in terms of squeezing, cramping, or pressure.

30. D: Fentanyl is a potent opioid medication that is available in a transdermal patch. Analgesic effects of the fentanyl patch last about 72 hours, but steady-state serum fentanyl levels are not reached until at least 12 hours after patch placement. Transdermal fentanyl is a useful analgesic tool for the palliative care patient with chronic, stable pain who is unable to take oral medications or experiences intolerable adverse effects with oral narcotics. Transdermal fentanyl is appropriate for the palliative care patient who is already tolerant to comparably potent opioids; it is not for use in patients who are just starting opiate medication for pain control. Transdermal fentanyl has a slow onset and offset, which makes it ineffective and inappropriate for treatment of breakthrough or incident pain, or for treatment of poorly controlled pain.

31. B: Pruritus, a persistent, unpleasant itching sensation, is common in the palliative care patient and may arise from a variety of causes (e.g., paraneoplastic, drug-related, caused by rash). Assessment should include a thorough evaluation of possible etiology, location, and quality, presence or absence of skin changes, and exacerbating or alleviating factors. Treatment should be tailored, if possible, to the specific cause of pruritus. If the skin is intact in affected areas, general principles of treatment include avoidance of heat or other exacerbating factors, application of topical moisturizers, and avoidance of further irritation by rubbing or scratching.

32. C: Terminal restlessness (also called terminal delirium or terminal agitation) is observed in a significant percentage of dying patients and can be very distressing to the patient's loved ones, who usually perceive the symptoms as a sign of suffering. Terminal restlessness may include moaning, crying out, hallucinating, tossing and turning, trying to get out of bed, and twitching. As with other episodes of delirium, an underlying cause (e.g., urinary retention, pain, medication effect) should be explored and treated as appropriate. The palliative care nurse should support the patient and family through the symptoms of terminal restlessness. This includes education and reassurance, medication administration, and environmental comfort measures.

33. B: Families often need a great deal of support and guidance in the hours immediately after death occurs. Though death often comes after a protracted illness, there can be unexpected emotional reactions once the death has actually occurred. Loved ones should be encouraged to spend time with the deceased, to perform any spiritual or personal rituals that are important to them, and to have physical contact with the deceased if they feel comfortable. If there is medical equipment (e.g., catheters, infusion pumps) that is interfering with the family's ability to spend time with the patient, the nurse should remove it. Families often appreciate assistance with arranging transfer to the funeral home and should be supported through the process of removing the body from the home. Family members may wish to bathe the patient before the body is taken from the home; the nurse should ask loved ones if they would like to participate in bathing the patient after death occurs.

34. D: The palliative care nurse may be faced with patient caregivers who are under- or overconfident in their ability to care for their loved one at the end of life. The nurse should assess each caregiver's coping and learning styles and fund of existing knowledge and comfort, and adjust both the tone and content of caregiver education accordingly. For the caregiver who appears overconfident in his or her knowledge base, the nurse should acknowledge the caregiver's comfort and knowledge while ensuring that family members are taught the specific information and skills necessary for maximizing the comfort of each particular patient. Condescension is not a compassionate or helpful communication technique.

35. D: The most important aspect of analgesic titration is repeated assessment of the patient's response to changes in the medication regimen. In this patient, it is most appropriate to calculate his consistent immediate-release morphine requirements (in mg), divide the total into two doses, and increase the dosage of his sustained-release morphine accordingly. If the patient's breakthrough pain is inconsistent or incident-related, it would be appropriate to continue the current regimen. If the patient's pain returns before the next scheduled dose of immediate-release morphine, it would be appropriate to decrease the interval between doses. If the patient's breakthrough pain is not adequately treated with the current dose of immediate-release morphine, it would be appropriate to increase the dose of the immediate-release opioid.

36. B: Symptoms of hypercalcemia are nonspecific and may be mistakenly attributed to the palliative care patient's underlying disease. Hypercalcemia causes gastrointestinal symptoms (e.g., nausea, vomiting, anorexia, constipation), neurological symptoms (e.g., fatigue, weakness, confusion), and cardiac symptoms. Hypoglycemia typically causes agitation, diaphoresis, and seizures. Hyponatremia causes primarily neurological symptoms, such as lethargy and weakness. Hypocalcemia causes paresthesias, tetany, irritability, and seizures.

37. C: Malodorous wounds can create a great deal of distress for patients and can interfere with patients' social functioning and dignity. The most common cause of wound odor is anaerobic bacterial colonization. Treatment strategies for both preventing and managing wound odor include frequent debridement and wound cleaning (as tolerated), application of topical metronidazole, and the use of charcoal dressings or charcoal in the patient's room. Charcoal is an effective odor-absorbing agent when dry. Once saturated, charcoal is no longer effective for odor reduction. Silver nitrate may be indicated for control of wound bleeding, but is not useful for management of wound odor.

38. D: Superior vena cava (SVC) syndrome is caused by obstruction of blood flow through the superior vena cava, most commonly by tumor compression (e.g., lung cancer, mediastinal lymphadenopathy) or a clot in the SVC. The most common symptom of SVC syndrome is shortness of breath. Other signs and symptoms include facial/arm/neck swelling, ruddy facial coloring, respiratory distress (e.g., stridor, tachypnea), distended neck veins, and dysphagia. If SVC obstruction comes on rapidly or is complete, the patient deteriorates rapidly because of increased intracranial pressure.

39. C: The Medicare Hospice Benefit is a federal program for Medicare-eligible patients with an estimated life expectancy of 6 months or less. Room and board, treatments or medications used with intent to cure, and hospice care from a different provider than originally designated, are not covered under the Medicare Hospice Benefit. Provider services (e.g., physician, nurse, social worker, and home health aide), supplies and equipment related to treatment of the terminal illness, and patient/family grief support are all covered. Medications (for symptom relief) and short-term respite care may require copay but are also covered under the Medicare Hospice Benefit.

40. A: Effective pain management depends on repeated and accurate pain assessment in the palliative care patient. Pain assessment should be performed when a patient is first evaluated by the palliative care team or admitted to a hospice facility. Pain assessments are also indicated at appropriate regular intervals if the patient is reporting pain; after administration of analgesic medication or other pain-management interventions; when the pain management plan has been changed; and when the patient is reporting a new type of pain. If a pain assessment is not consistent with the patient's end-of-life goals, or if the patient declines, a pain assessment is not appropriate unless there are other compelling factors present.

41. C: Morphine remains one of the most commonly used opioid analgesics in palliative care and may be administered to the patient via multiple possible routes. The IV (parenteral) route of administration provides the fastest time to onset of analgesia (usually within 1-3 minutes). Onset of analgesic effect for subcutaneous or intramuscular administration is typically 10-30 minutes after administration. Oral or rectal administration leads to onset of analgesic effect 30-60 minutes after administration. In general, oral administration of pain medication is the delivery method of choice for the palliative care patient, although alternate routes may be necessary as death approaches or as dictated by the patient's clinical condition.

42. C: Signs of impending death in the palliative care patient (e.g., decreased level of consciousness, decreased food/fluid intake, increased heart rate, and decreased urine output) typically appear somewhat gradually over the course of days or even weeks when associated with progression of the underlying illness. When these signs develop acutely (e.g., over the course of several hours), they may be indicative of a potentially reversible cause of deterioration, such as infection or electrolyte abnormalities. The patient's medications should also be reviewed when deterioration occurs rapidly; changes in medication or dosages may result in improvement. Not all acute causes of deterioration would necessarily be indications for treatment, depending on the patient's specific end-of-life goals.

43. D: Intrathecal infusion of morphine, bupivacaine, and/or clonidine may be used for pain management in patients with intractable pain who are not responsive to other analgesic regimens. Nurses caring for patients receiving intrathecal analgesia need to be familiar with care of the catheter, signs and symptoms of intrathecal analgesia complications, and emergency management of complications. Hypotension may occur with infusion of local anesthetic medication (e.g., bupivacaine) as a result of vasodilation secondary to sympathetic nerve block. The patient may report feeling "faint," lightheaded, or dizzy. Management of hypotension includes IV fluid administration and IV ephedrine administration as needed for significant hypotension. Other possible complications of intrathecal analgesia are catheter dislodgement, infection, cerebrospinal fluid leak, urinary retention, muscle weakness, and respiratory depression (due to either narcotic-mediated respiratory depression or diaphragmatic weakness due to local anesthetic).

44. A: Helping patients maintain hope in the face of terminal illness and impending death is an important tool of the palliative care nurse. Hope is a healthy and adaptive response to life, even in the setting of life-threatening illness. Hope arises from a variety of sources, including meaningful relationships, fun, feeling worthwhile, and aiming for both short- and long-term goals. Nurses can help patients maintain hope at the end of life in numerous ways, including managing distressing physical symptoms, using humor as appropriate, encouraging activities that the patient enjoys, encouraging positive self-talk, helping patients set end-of-life goals, and providing straightforward information about the patient's disease and treatment.

45. D: The International Association for Hospice and Palliative Care describes palliative care as "the care of patients with active, progressive, far-advanced disease for whom the focus of care is the relief and prevention of suffering and the quality of life." A common misconception among patients and healthcare providers is that palliative care consultation should only be sought after all standard medical therapeutic options for the patient's disease(s) have failed. The palliative care team's emphasis on the whole patient (including psychosocial, cultural, and spiritual sources of strength or distress) can be extremely helpful with symptom relief, prioritization of therapeutic options, choice of care setting, patient and family peace of mind, and numerous other issues. A patient with disease in remission is not a good candidate for palliative care consultation.

46. A: Corticosteroids may be used to treat a variety of conditions and symptoms in the palliative care patient, including cerebral edema, spinal cord compression, pain, nausea/vomiting, malignant bowel obstruction, fatigue, and loss of appetite. Although steroids can be very effective, they are associated with frequent and significant adverse effects, particularly with prolonged use. Common effects of even short-term steroid use include disturbed sleep, hyperglycemia, delirium or agitation, fluid retention, gastric ulceration, and increased susceptibility to infection. Prolonged steroid use may lead to osteoporosis, myopathy, and cataracts.

47. D: Parkinson's disease is a common, progressive neurodegenerative disease characterized by bradykinesia (slowed movement), resting tremor, rigidity, and disturbances in gait, posture, and balance. Patients in the later stages of Parkinson's disease experience less benefit from medications used to treat the symptoms of the disease. Late-stage Parkinson's disease is associated with marked impairment in communication, ambulation, and cognition in most patients. Common signs and symptoms include memory loss, hallucinations, agitation, severe depression, difficulty swallowing (leading to weight loss), difficulty speaking, pain, inability to walk, drooling, incontinence, and severe rigidity and bradykinesia.

48. A: Nausea and vomiting are a common adverse effect of opioid administration, regardless of the route of administration. Nausea and vomiting due to opioid use are most pronounced in the first few days after starting the medication, and often decrease over time. Although cannabinoids may be a useful adjunct in treating nausea and vomiting, they are not recommended as first-line agents. Opioid-associated nausea may respond to a variety of medications, including haloperidol, metoclopramide, and ondansetron. If nausea and vomiting persist after several days of opioid use, it may be helpful to change to a different opioid medication. It is also important to ensure that the patient is not experiencing nausea and vomiting secondary to opioid-related constipation.

49. C: Constipation with associated stool impaction may lead to leakage of liquid stool around impacted solid stool. Appropriate constipation management, including disimpaction if necessary, will lead to resolution of overflow incontinence. Stool leakage is often very upsetting and embarrassing to patients and can lead to physical complications, such as perineal skin breakdown, as well as psychosocial complications, such as loss of dignity or social isolation. Secretory diarrhea in the palliative care patient may be caused by cancer treatment or paraneoplastic conditions, and is characterized by very large volumes of liquid stool production. Hypercalcemia is more likely to cause constipation than diarrhea. Diarrhea in association with acute infectious enteritis is usually associated with abdominal cramping and may also be guaiac-positive or grossly bloody.

50. B: Worry and sadness are appropriate, expected reactions to the challenge of life-threatening disease and all the life changes that accompany serious illness. If a patient's anxiety and sadness are persistent, unrelenting, or severe, the patient would likely benefit from psychiatric evaluation and treatment. Although prior mental health and coping skills are highly predictive of the patient's ability to adjust psychologically to life-threatening illness, the diagnosis of anxiety or depressive disorder does not depend on the patient's psychiatric history. Severity of disease and life expectancy are not necessarily related to the patient's psychological reaction to illness.

51. A: For adequate symptom management at the end of life, most terminally ill patients will require medications with addiction and abuse potential (e.g., opiates, benzodiazepines). Past or current drug addiction can pose difficult challenges for both patients and providers in the setting of terminal illness. For the terminally ill patient with an addiction problem, general principles of pain management include ensuring consistent practice among all members of the care team, monitoring for addiction behaviors, maximizing the use of adjuvant analgesic therapies and sustained-release opiates (rather than immediate-release), and maintaining a commitment to treat pain and suffering, even in the patient whose drug addiction complicates pain assessment and management. In most patients with active addiction issues, small supplies of opiate medications should be prescribed at a time to discourage drug diversion, and frequent evaluation and follow-up with the care team should be encouraged.

52. A: A child's perception of death is highly dependent on his or her developmental stage. During life-threatening illness and after the death of a loved one, children should receive age-appropriate, direct communication from the adults in their lives. Overt expressions of grief such as crying or acting out are often intermittent in children, interspersed with play and happy times. Maintaining important routines is valuable and therapeutic for the grieving child. Children should be encouraged to express all of their feelings and to remember the deceased in ways that are appropriate and meaningful to them.

53. A: Oral administration is the route of choice for opioid medications in the palliative care patient, but most patients require an alternative route of administration at some point in their illness. Opioids are available in oral, rectal, sublingual, transdermal, intravenous, subcutaneous, intraspinal, intranasal, and topical formulations. Rectal opioids are easy to administer, are available in immediate- or sustained-release formulations, and are readily prepared in virtually any dosage strength. Opioids administered rectally are absorbed into the systemic circulation through the rectal veins. Absorption is largely independent of GI tract functioning or motility, making rectal opioids an excellent choice in patients with vomiting, bowel obstruction, or malabsorption. Because of variations in the vascular supply and possible interference with constipation or stooling, rectal opioid absorption may be highly variable.

54. A: The provision of artificial nutrition and hydration in the terminally ill patient remains a muddy and controversial issue in palliative care. The expected decrease in oral intake associated with progressive terminal illness is not usually associated with feelings of thirst or hunger and is often far more upsetting to the patient's loved ones than to the patient. If the patient's decrease in appetite is due to poorly controlled symptoms (e.g., pain, hiccups, constipation, nausea), improved management of the symptoms that are causing suffering will likely lead to improved appetite. If the patient is distressed by the degree of anorexia, further intervention may be warranted (e.g., steroids). Tube feeding should only be used with the goal of meeting specific end-of-life goals (e.g., increased energy) in accordance with the patient's priorities.

55. B: Alternative routes to oral, enteral, and IV fluid administration in the palliative care patient include proctoclysis (rectally administered) and hypodermoclysis (subcutaneously administered). Hypodermoclysis consists of placing and securing a butterfly needle or angiocatheter in the subcutaneous space, which is used for bolus or continuous fluid administration with standard tubing and IV fluids. Advantages of subcutaneous fluid administration include less discomfort with placement, easier catheter placement, and a wide variety of possible sites for catheter placement. These advantages make hypodermoclysis more appropriate for initiation and ongoing use in the home hospice setting. Unlike IV catheter use, there is no concern for intravascular clot or air embolus with a subcutaneous catheter.

56. D: Durable medical equipment (DME) or home medical equipment required for care of the patient's terminal illness is 100% covered under the Medicare Hospice Benefit. This includes delivery and maintenance of the necessary supplies, as well as training on their use. Common supplies that qualify as DME are commodes, walkers, oxygen, infusion pumps, and hospital beds. Although it can be demoralizing for some patients to recognize that their illness has progressed to the point of needing medical equipment in their home, durable medical equipment helps enable patients to maintain their independence and dignity.

57. A: Dysphagia is common in palliative care patients, and may arise from cognitive impairment, weakness, mechanical obstruction, incoordination, and medications. Although dietary modifications such as pureed food or thickened liquid are helpful for many patients with dysphagia, there are other strategies for managing dysphagia in the patient who wants to continue eating. Chilled food, postural adjustment (e.g., chin tuck, head tilt), and deliberate swallowing awareness are helpful for many patients with dysphagia.

58. C: Tricyclic antidepressants, such as amitriptyline, are effective for treating neuropathic pain (in doses lower than those required for antidepressant effect), but adverse effects are common and may limit their use. This patient's constellation of symptoms is consistent with the anticholinergic effects of tricyclic antidepressants (dry mouth, urinary retention, delirium, tachycardia, constipation, and blurry vision). Other adverse effects include cardiac arrhythmia, sexual dysfunction, weight gain, perspiration, orthostatic hypotension, and sedation.

59. C: Selecting the appropriate analgesic medication and route depends on an accurate and thorough pain assessment. Characterizing the nature of a patient's pain allows the provider to select an effective analgesic while minimizing toxicity or adverse effects. Breakthrough pain refers to intermittent episodes of moderate to severe pain that typically come on rapidly and are relatively short-lasting. Given the nature of breakthrough pain, a rapid-onset and shorter-acting analgesic administered as needed is most appropriate for treatment. The oral route is generally preferred for administration of pain medications in the palliative care patient, although each patient's clinical status and progression must take precedence over general guidelines.

60. A: Constipation is a common problem in the palliative care patient because of a variety of factors that increase the likelihood of constipation, such as opiate (and other) medications, decreased mobility, poor oral fluid intake, metabolic derangements (e.g., hypercalcemia), mechanical obstruction to abdominal tumors, and spinal cord compression. Constipation may lead to agitation, abdominal pain, urinary retention or incontinence, and overflow liquid stool leakage. Fever is not caused by constipation alone; if fever is present, the patient should be assessed (as appropriate) for an infectious source.

61. B: Although some families do respond to the illness of a loved one with cooperation and improved communication, it is unrealistic to expect a stressed and challenged family to successfully tackle years of dysfunctional family dynamics in the context of life-threatening illness. Assessment of family dynamics over time allows the palliative care team to appropriately individualize support and communication interventions in the context of terminal illness. In families that lack open lines of communication among family members, the palliative care nurse should expect to communicate important information to family members individually to ensure that the information is imparted effectively and consistently.

62. D: Nausea is a frequent adverse effect of opioid medication and is primarily caused by central nervous system effects and impaired gastrointestinal motility. The drug of choice for opioid-related nausea is haloperidol. The dosage used for nausea is lower than the typical antipsychotic dosing, resulting in a lower incidence of extrapyramidal and sedative adverse effects. 5-HT3 receptor antagonists (e.g., ondansetron) are also effective and may work especially well when combined with haloperidol. Although prokinetic agents, such as metoclopramide, may be indicated in patients with a component of decreased gastric motility, they are not first-line antiemetics. Dexamethasone has some antiemetic properties but is not the therapy of choice in this case, and naloxone is rarely indicated in the palliative care patient because of the risk of precipitating a pain crisis.

63. A: It is critically important for the palliative care nurse to be aware of the relative potencies of different opioids and to understand how to calculate equianalgesic doses when changing from one opioid to another. The process of converting from one opioid to another begins with a calculation of the total 24-hour dose of the current medication. Morphine is the medication that all other opioids are compared with for the purpose of equianalgesic calculations. Therefore, if the original medication is not morphine, the 24-hour dosage total should be converted to an equianalgesic dose of morphine. The 24-hour morphine dose can then be converted (using the medication and route-specific conversion factor) to an equianalgesic dose of the new medication. If the pain is well controlled with the old medication, the provider may reduce the equianalgesic dose of the new medication by 25-50% to begin with. With this example, oxycodone is approximately twice as potent as oral morphine; in other words, oral morphine 20 mg is equivalent to oral oxycodone 10 mg. It is not appropriate to continue the original opioid when changing to a different medication because of the risk of toxicity due to excessive narcotic administration.

64. C: Regardless of the primary disease, the dying process is remarkably similar in most patients who are dying of a chronic illness. Dying patients become less aware of their surroundings and have a reduced desire or ability to move around. Breathing is often noisy because of pooling oral secretions (i.e., the "death rattle") and the respiratory pattern may be irregular. Urine output drops precipitously or stops altogether. As death approaches, circulation and oxygenation are impaired, leading to cool, mottled extremities. The palliative care nurse should be familiar with the common signs and symptoms of impending death so that he or she can educate and support the patient and family members during the dying process.

65. C: Palliative sedation refers to the administration of sedative medication (e.g., benzodiazepines) to the terminally ill patient for the purpose of relieving severe, intractable symptoms that are causing suffering. The most common indications are intractable agitation, dyspnea, or pain. Palliative sedation is indicated only when all other reasonable therapies for the patient's severe symptoms have been ineffective. Other comfort measures should not be discontinued in the patient receiving palliative sedation, although monitoring and therapy that is not aimed at increasing patient comfort should be stopped. Palliative sedation remains somewhat controversial. Some believe that it represents the ethical equivalent of euthanasia because of the possibility of hastened death when sedatives are titrated to relieve patient suffering. Honest and thorough discussions between the patient, family members, and care providers (including the nurse) are extremely important before the decision is made to use palliative sedation.

66. B: Spiritual pain is a very real and painful phenomenon in some palliative care patients. It may arise from various sources, including guilt or grief about past events, distress over the loss of independence or dignity at the end of life, fears or loss of hope regarding death, and religious or faith concerns. Spiritual pain may manifest itself in a variety of ways, including physical pain that is unresponsive to appropriate therapy, interpersonal conflicts, anger, anxiety, hopelessness, and refusal of medication. Helpful interventions will depend on the patient's individual perspective and beliefs, making multidimensional pain assessment crucial for these patients. When first learning of a patient's spiritual distress, the palliative care nurse should listen actively and gently attempt to elicit more information from the patient to further flesh out the contributing factors to the patient's spiritual pain. It is the patient's belief system that should guide therapeutic intervention, not the nurse's.

67. C: Though anorexia and cachexia are commonly present in terminally ill patients, they are distinct conditions. Anorexia is characterized by loss of appetite that leads to decreased nutritional intake and weight loss. Anorexia (or starvation) leads to decreased energy expenditure and loss of primarily adipose (fat) tissue rather than lean muscle mass. The weight loss associated with anorexia is reversible with improved nutritional intake. Cachexia is a multisystem condition caused by a systemic inflammatory response and is associated with increased energy expenditure, equal loss of fat and lean muscle, fatigue, anemia, and decreased immune function. The weight loss associated with cachexia is not reversed with nutritional supplementation.

68. A: Delirium is a common phenomenon in the palliative care patient and may be caused by the patient's underlying illness, medications, and/or environmental factors. Antipsychotics (usually haloperidol) are the treatment of choice for most cases of delirium, assuming that a reversible etiology has not been identified. Benzodiazepines (such as lorazepam) commonly cause increased agitation when used alone for the treatment of delirium (though they are the treatment of choice for delirium caused by drug or alcohol withdrawal).

69. D: Withholding artificial hydration and/or nutrition in the terminally ill patient is very distressing for many families and can be difficult for many providers as well. In the United States, artificial hydration is considered a medical intervention, and its use can therefore be refused if the patient and/or care team feel its burdens outweigh the benefits. Artificial hydration may exacerbate end-of-life symptoms, including vomiting, edema, and respiratory secretions. In addition, the equipment required for artificial hydration may cause discomfort or make it more difficult for patients to have unencumbered physical contact with loved ones.

70. B: There are numerous potential barriers to the provision of high-quality palliative care for the patient living in poverty. A patient may be viewed as noncompliant or difficult when he or she is having difficulty establishing trust with the palliative care team or having difficulty accessing adequate medical care because of a lack of transportation, housing, or financial resources. Although it may be appropriate in some cases to advise patients to use personal financial resources or to spend time advocating for themselves with insurance providers, the most appropriate action in this case is for the nurse to help the patient access a medication that will be covered by Medicaid.

71. A: Providing effective spiritual support to the palliative care patient begins with the palliative care provider exploring and gaining comfort with his or her own spiritual beliefs and challenges. Though there may be significant difference between patient and provider in religious and spiritual beliefs or practices, the self-aware nurse can provide a great deal of spiritual support to patients at the end of life. The most important intervention in most cases is a compassionate and empathetic presence. Active listening creates a safe, nonjudgmental environment for the patient to express and process spiritual challenges, concerns, and crises.

72. C: While the palliative care nurse will hopefully end up discovering answers to all of the above questions (and more), certain questions can help both the patient and the nurse clarify the specific quality-of-life priorities that should guide the plan of care. For example, questions such as "What symptoms bother you most?" or "How has your illness interfered with your daily life?" or "What are your priorities in terms of quality of life versus duration of life?" can assist the provider in symptom management and in formulating a plan of care that is consistent with the patient's wishes.

73. C: Pooling of upper respiratory tract secretions is common in the dying patient and leads to the so-called "death rattle." Most patients exhibiting this sort of respiratory congestion are not suffering or in pain, although loved ones are usually very distressed by the patient's breathing. Nonpharmacologic measures include repositioning, avoiding overhydration, and compassionately educating and reassuring the patient's loved ones. Available pharmacologic treatment options consist of anticholinergic agents that decrease secretions, such as hyoscine hydrobromide, atropine sulfate, and glycopyrrolate.

74. D: Myoclonus in the palliative care patient is most commonly caused by opiate medications, usually in association with prolonged and/or high-dose opioid administration. Myoclonic movements are involuntary, sudden, brief jerking movements usually involving the extremities. Unlike seizures, myoclonus does not cause impairment in the patient's level of consciousness or responsiveness. Myoclonus is often very distressing (and exhausting) to patients. Myoclonus is considered a sign of opiate toxicity and is an indication for switching to a different opioid agent. Treatment of severe myoclonus may include benzodiazepine or antispasmodic administration (in addition to discontinuation of the offending opioid agent).

75. B: Numerous barriers get in the way of adequate pain relief in the palliative care patient, many of which originate with patients themselves. Common patient factors that interfere with adequate pain assessment and treatment are fear of addiction, fatalistic attitudes about pain, concerns about analgesic adverse effects, fear that pain indicates worsening disease, and sociocultural beliefs about stoicism. Eliciting the patient's knowledge, beliefs, and misconceptions about pain is crucial so that patient-related barriers to pain management can be minimized through education and counseling. If the nurse helps the patient to see that his or her preferences and goals for end-of-life care can be more effectively addressed if all symptoms are accurately reported, this is usually more effective than directly challenging a deeply held social or cultural belief about pain.

76. A: Patients and caregivers need careful instructions for proper use of the transdermal fentanyl patch to avoid complications of excessive opioid effect or inadequate pain control. The fentanyl patch should be placed over intact skin in a hairless region (if possible) and should be changed every 72 hours in most patients. Heat applied over the patch (or increased body temperature due to fever) may increase the rate of fentanyl absorption, and should therefore be avoided. Used patches still contain a significant amount of fentanyl, and accidental ingestion by other members of the household may result in life-threatening overdose. Patches should therefore be folded with adhesive surfaces stuck together and either flushed down the toilet immediately or discarded in a location safe from pets and children. Patients experiencing breakthrough pain despite use of the fentanyl patch may still take as-needed opiate doses via alternate routes of administration.

77. D: Brain and spinal complications and metastases are common with many malignancies, particularly cancers of the lung, breast, prostate, myeloma, and melanoma. Brain metastases typically present with unilateral neurological deficits (e.g., weakness, sensory changes, cranial nerve palsies), headache, altered mental status, and seizures. In contrast, spinal metastases typically present with back pain, extremity weakness (may be asymmetric but is often bilateral), extremity paresthesias/sensory changes, and autonomic dysfunction manifested by urinary and/or bowel retention or incontinence. Degenerative arthritis commonly causes back pain but would not typically be associated with this patient's other symptoms, and would be far less likely than spinal metastatic disease in a young patient with melanoma.

78. B: It is widely believed that, in most dying patients, the last sense to be lost is hearing. This is based in part on firsthand reports from patients who have been in a comatose state and later recalled sounds and statements that were made while they were comatose. Visual acuity decreases as a patient approaches death, and visual disturbances (e.g., illusions, hallucinations) are common. The patient's family members should be taught that their dying loved one can likely hear what is going on around them long after he or she is able to respond. Caregivers often find great comfort knowing that their dying loved one can hear what people are saying to them, and patients may be calmed with familiar music or voices.

79. B: The palliative care nurse should be comfortable using widely available opioid conversion charts. Patients may be changing administration route for the same medication, changing the medication while using the same route of administration, or changing both medication and route of administration. This patient is changing from parenteral morphine to oral morphine. The conversion rate between parenteral and oral morphine is 1:3. Therefore, intravenous morphine 1 mg is equivalent to oral morphine 3 mg. The patient's total intravenous morphine dose over 24 hours is 30 mg. Multiplying 30 × 3 (the conversion rate from intravenous to oral) equals 90 mg. This is the 24-hour total dose of oral morphine. Dividing this by 2 (for twice-daily administration) results in an oral regimen of sustained-release oral morphine 45 mg twice daily.

80. D: The Medicare Hospice Benefit is a federal program for Medicare-eligible patients (of any age) with an estimated life expectancy of 6 months or less. Eligibility requirements do not vary from state to state. A "do not resuscitate" (DNR) order is not required for eligibility, but the patient must opt out of "regular" Medicare (Part A) in order to be covered under the Medicare Hospice Benefit. Physician care, nursing care, medications, and supplies are covered under the Medicare Hospice Benefit, and hospice care may be provided in multiple settings (e.g., home, inpatient, and outpatient).

81. C: Effects of dehydration include fewer respiratory secretions, lower urine output/incontinence, less vomiting and diarrhea, less interstitial fluid (e.g., ascites, pleural effusions), and increased risk of pressure injuries, constipation, and thirst. Decreased renal function caused by dehydration leads to more drug and metabolite accumulation. Depending on the individual patient, the effects of dehydration may be beneficial in managing end-of-life symptoms or, conversely, may increase uncomfortable or unpleasant symptoms. End-of-life symptoms that arise from dehydration should be managed in accordance with the patient's goals and wishes.

82. B: There are numerous barriers to the provision of optimal palliative care in the elderly population because of a variety of factors. Predicting limited life spans in the setting of nonmalignant chronic diseases, such as heart failure or dementia, is difficult. This leads to underutilization of hospice services available to elderly patients. Many elderly patients have impaired cognition and/or expressive communication, making it challenging for care providers to assess pain and other forms of distress. In addition, age-related factors, such as reduced liver function or changes in body composition, lead to increased potential for medication complications. Most nursing homes do not provide adequate palliative care to their elderly residents because of a lack of staff awareness, education, and nurse/physician availability. All patients have the right to make independent and well-informed choices about end-of-life care, and research has repeatedly demonstrated that patients prefer to be asked about these issues. Generally, it is family members and medical providers, not patients themselves, who are hesitant to initiate a conversation about end-of-life issues.

83. D: Conveying "bad news" compassionately and truthfully is an important skill for palliative care providers, including nurses. As with other aspects of palliative care, the patient's wishes and priorities should be respected. It is appropriate and reasonable for patients to delay hearing details about a diagnosis or prognosis until they feel that they have the support and emotional resources to deal with the conversation. If there is demonstrated harm caused by the patient's lack of readiness to hear all of the relevant clinical information, supportive and gentle intervention may be warranted.

84. A: Prevention of pressure injuries in the inactive or immobile palliative care patient depends on identification of risk factors and prevention techniques. Use of a number of strategies, depending on the patient's particular risk factors and plan of care, is warranted. These generally include passive repositioning, pillow-bridging, pressure-relieving support surfaces, avoidance of friction and shear trauma, moisture management, and nutritional support. Passive repositioning by the patient's caregiver should be done on a schedule to avoid inadvertently allowing long periods of immobility. Full-body passive repositioning should be provided approximately every 2 hours to minimize risk of pressure injuries.

85. B: "Titration to effect" refers to the increase or decrease in analgesic dosing based on the patient's reported pain severity and the patient's responses to changes in dose. Titration may include increased dosage amount or frequency. Ideally, analgesic medication is titrated to the dose that allows for adequate pain control with minimal adverse effects. Adverse effects do not necessarily preclude further dosage increases; other strategies for managing adverse effects of analgesic medications may allow for further dosage increases as needed for better pain management. The patient's reported severity of pain should dictate dose adjustments. Many patients do not appear to an outside observer to be in pain, when they are actually experiencing significant discomfort.

86. B: Corticosteroids may be used to treat a variety of conditions and symptoms that are present in the palliative care patient. One of the most common uses for steroids in palliative care is treatment of symptoms related to central nervous system malignancy and metastatic disease. These include headache, seizure, confusion, spinal cord compression, asymptomatic brain tumor edema, and focal neurological deficits. Other common indications in the palliative care patient include pain due to bony metastases, anorexia and fatigue, neuropathic pain, visceral pain, dyspnea secondary to lung or airway inflammation, and vomiting. Less commonly, steroids may also be used for the treatment of hypercalcemia, neoplastic fever, and malignant bowel obstruction. Delirium is a possible adverse effect of steroid administration.

87. C: The phenomenon of an apparent awareness or expression of readiness for approaching death is referred to as nearing death awareness (NDA) and is frequently observed in the dying patient. NDA may manifest as a description of a journey or visions of deceased loved ones or a spiritual being. It may be difficult to distinguish between NDA and delirium or agitation. If the patient does not appear uncomfortable or upset as he or she makes seemingly confused statements, the best action is to listen and affirm the patient's experience. It is not helpful to try to forcefully orient the patient or dispute what he or she is reporting. Sedatives are not indicated if the patient's experience seems to be more consistent with NDA than agitation or delirium.

88. A: Carcinoid tumors typically arise in the intestinal tract and can be benign. Larger carcinoid tumors frequently metastasize to the liver and may cause carcinoid syndrome, a paraneoplastic complication due to elevated levels of hormones that are secreted by the tumor. Carcinoid tumors may secrete a variety of hormones, including histamine, serotonin, and catecholamines. Clinical manifestations are determined by the specific hormones secreted by the tumor. Common symptoms of carcinoid syndrome include diarrhea, flushing, abdominal cramping, wheezing, right heart failure, and cyanosis. Treatment may include symptomatic therapy (e.g., diuretics, bronchodilators), tumor debulking, and medications that block hormonal secretion (e.g., somatostatin analogues, such as octreotide).

89. A: Diarrhea is an extremely challenging and unpleasant symptom for the palliative care patient and may lead to psychosocial and physical complications (e.g., loss of dignity, skin breakdown, dehydration). After assessment and treatment of the underlying cause of the patient's diarrhea, nursing interventions include attention to environmental management, hydration, skin care, and psychosocial support. Many patients are resistant to wearing diapers, and there are environmental strategies that allow the patient's preference to be honored. This may entail removing physical obstacles to the toilet, assisting with moving the patient to the commode or toilet, and placing protective materials (e.g., Chux) under the patient. Meticulous skin care with barrier cream and increased oral fluid intake (as tolerated) are important supportive measures in the patient with diarrhea.

90. A: Spinal cord compression requires emergent recognition and intervention to prevent permanent neurological disability. In the palliative care patient, spinal cord compression is most commonly associated with vertebral metastases of breast, prostate, and lung cancers. The most common presenting symptom of spinal cord compression is back pain, which is worse when lying flat or straining (e.g., coughing, stooling) and improves upon standing. Other symptoms that develop as compression worsens include weakness, sensory changes, and bowel and bladder dysfunction.

91. B: Delirium is an acute and fluctuating state characterized by disordered attention, cognition, perception, and level of consciousness. Supportive and environmental measures can greatly reduce the patient's agitation and improve the symptoms of delirium. Maintaining a familiar environment with known sounds, smells, textures, and care providers is important. Avoiding isolation or overstimulation and providing gentle repeated reassurance can be helpful. Maintaining cues of day and night, such as natural light, may improve sleep disturbance.

92. D: Many patients require controlled substances (e.g., opiates, benzodiazepines) for symptom management at the end of life. Safe storage of these potent medications while the patient is taking them is paramount. Controlled substances should be kept out of the reach of children, strangers, loved ones with a prior or current addiction problem, and pets. When the patient has died or no longer requires the medication, federal regulations dictate that hospice agencies must have a policy for the disposal of controlled substances. This may involve discussing proper disposal techniques with family caregivers, assisting the family with proper disposal, and notifying the dispensing pharmacists that refills are no longer authorized.

93. B: Patients facing a terminal illness often experience spiritual or existential distress, which may be related to their perception of the value or meaning of their lives, unresolved conflicts with loved ones, unwelcome changes in their lives brought on by illness, and crises of religious or spiritual faith. The palliative care nurse can assist the patient in achieving "self-determined life closure" and finding meaning in life and death by encouraging the patient to perform a life review. This essentially entails encouraging and listening as the patient shares his or her life story. Often, life review helps patients identify the experiences and people that have been most important in their lives, find peace and forgiveness in past conflicts and challenges, recognize the value in their lives, and see the meaningful connections between the past and the present.

94. D: Communication with patients about benefits versus burdens of therapeutic interventions requires an ability to provide accurate information in a manner that helps the patient make a decision within the framework of his or her goals and priorities for end-of-life care. For example, a patient who hopes to live long enough to participate in a certain family event may opt for therapeutic interventions that are most likely to prolong duration of life, even at the expense of quality of life. Any conversation about the benefits versus burdens of a therapeutic intervention should include anticipated benefits to the patient, anticipated complications or disadvantages, anticipated effect (if any) on both duration and quality of life, and how all of these apply to the patient's individual priorities and goals. Patients always retain the right to change their mind with regard to either initiating or stopping a therapeutic intervention.

95. B: Anticholinergic medications (e.g., oxybutynin) are a common adjunct for management of urinary incontinence because of their inhibitory effect on bladder contractility. The most common adverse effect associated with anticholinergic medication is dry mouth, which may lead to oral complications in the palliative care patient. Other adverse effects of anticholinergic medications include constipation, blurry vision, fatigue, flushing, and tachycardia.

96. D: Fever is a common symptom in the palliative care patient and can cause a great deal of discomfort to patients. In addition to antipyretic medications (e.g., acetaminophen), general comfort measures include changing moist clothes and linens, oral care, maintenance of comfortable room temperature, skin care, and oral fluids or ice chips for thirst. Although gentle cooling measures (e.g., lukewarm moist cloth on the forehead) may increase patient comfort, aggressive cooling (e.g., ice baths, cooling blankets) is often uncomfortable and may increase heat production by causing the patient to shiver.

97. D: Relative contraindications to the use of NSAIDs for the treatment of pain in the palliative care patient include renal or liver dysfunction, gastrointestinal bleeding, and platelet dysfunction/thrombocytopenia. Pancreatic insufficiency is not a contraindication to NSAID use. Ibuprofen, aspirin, and naproxen are nonselective NSAIDs in that they inhibit both the COX-1 and COX-2 enzyme pathways affecting prostaglandin synthesis. Selective NSAIDs, such as celecoxib, act only on the COX-2 pathway, leading to decreased risk of gastrointestinal bleeding. Selective NSAIDs have been associated with increased risk of adverse cardiovascular events such as stroke and myocardial infarction.

98. A: The patient in this scenario has become bedbound as a result of terminal disease progression, a sign that death is likely in the near future. The most appropriate plan for addressing pressure injuries in this patient is palliative treatment, which meets the goal of maximum patient comfort rather than optimal wound healing. It is important for the palliative care nurse to recognize signs of impending death so that the patient and team of caregivers can continue to ensure that the patient's goals for end-of-life care remain the focus of treatment. As death approaches, unnecessarily invasive, painful, or disruptive treatments or monitoring devices should usually be discontinued. For most hospice patients in the terminal phase of illness, comfort and support are of primary importance.

99. A: Alcohol abuse and hepatitis B and C are the most common causes of cirrhosis in the United States. Complications of cirrhosis include coagulopathy, ascites, portal hypertension, hepatorenal syndrome, esophageal varices, and hepatic encephalopathy. Hepatic encephalopathy is characterized by personality changes, altered level of consciousness, and impairment in cognitive function. The pathophysiology of hepatic encephalopathy remains a topic of scientific research and debate, but in most patients with hepatic encephalopathy, serum ammonia levels are elevated and a fall in serum ammonia is associated with clinical improvement. The cirrhotic liver is not able to detoxify ammonia as well as the healthy liver does, leading to elevated serum ammonia levels. Any degree of portosystemic shunting of blood (common in many patients with cirrhosis) will also lead to elevated serum ammonia levels.

100. C: Lymphedema is caused by failure of adequate lymphatic drainage and most commonly affects the extremities. The affected extremity will be asymmetrically enlarged on examination. The patient often complains of skin tightness, blisters or weeping fluid, tingling, decreased range of motion, and possibly discomfort in the affected extremity. The mainstay of lymphedema therapy is external compression, which may be accomplished with bandages or particular compression garments. Frequent reevaluation and patience are required to find the compression device that is best tolerated by each patient. Management should also include surveillance and treatment of lymphedema complications (pain, infection), skin care, and healthy lifestyle habits (e.g., diet, appropriate exercise). Other therapeutic options include liposuction and diuretics.

101. D: Stool impaction increases the palliative care patient's risk of urinary retention, urinary incontinence, and urinary tract infection due to mechanical obstruction and urinary stasis. A thorough history and physical assessment in the patient with urinary tract disorders will usually reveal contributing factors. Addressing stool impaction will often lead to improvement or complete resolution of the patient's urinary symptoms. Hematuria is not a common complication of stool impaction and, if present, should be evaluated further (if appropriate within the patient's goals for end-of-life care).

102. D: Providing support and assistance for patients and families in preparing for death is one of the most important therapeutic interventions the palliative care nurse can provide. This entails teaching the patient and family about common symptoms as death approaches, assessing and managing psychic or physical suffering, supporting patients in the difficult discussions about goals for death and after-death services, and encouraging patients to identify the "last things" that are most important for them to accomplish.

103. C: Elder abuse is estimated to affect 1-2 million elderly adults annually and can take many different forms, including neglect, physical abuse, financial exploitation, and emotional abuse. Studies have demonstrated that male and female patients are equally likely to be victims of elder abuse. Risk of abuse also appears to be independent of race, socioeconomic status, and religious affiliation. Elderly adults are far more likely to be abused by family members (e.g., spouse, child) than nonfamily caregivers, and abuse is more likely to occur in the home setting. Caregivers with active mental illness and/or substance abuse are associated with increased risk of elder abuse. Patients with insufficient or dysfunctional social support systems are also at increased risk of abuse. There is insufficient or mixed data on other possible risk factors for elder abuse, such as caregiver stress level and cognitive impairment in the patient. The palliative care nurse should be proficient at identifying and responding to signs of elder abuse in the palliative care patient.

104. C: The initial certification of terminal illness for the first 90-day coverage period under the Medicare Hospice Benefit requires two-physician (the patient's primary physician and the hospice physician) certification that the patient's life expectancy is 6 months or less based on expected disease course, clinical information supporting the expected prognosis, and a brief narrative explanation of the clinical information. Initial recertification (covering an additional 90-day period) requires only the hospice physician to certify an anticipated life expectancy of 6 months or less with accompanying supportive clinical information and narrative. Hospice recertifications beyond the first 180-day coverage period (i.e., the third or later benefit period) require documentation of a face-to-face visit with the patient (by physician or nurse practitioner) that has the express purpose of gathering clinical information that supports the patient's continued hospice eligibility. This is in addition to physician certification of life expectancy 6 months or less with supportive clinical information and narrative. Malignancy is not a requirement for terminal illness certification.

105. A: Interdisciplinary collaboration refers to a group of people with complementary experience and expertise sharing decision-making, responsibility, and accountability in pursuit of a common goal. In the case of palliative care interdisciplinary collaboration, the goal is formulation of a care plan that meets the goals and preferences of the individual patient. Responsibility and accountability are shared, not diminished, among team members. In contrast to multidisciplinary teams, treatment decisions are made by the group, not by one member of the group. The challenges posed by interdisciplinary collaboration are those posed by any group process; differences in personality, professional culture, and comfort working in a group setting can make collaboration difficult depending on the team dynamics.

106. D: Xerostomia (the sensation of a dry mouth) is a common complaint in the palliative care patient and may lead to difficulty with chewing, swallowing, speaking, and taste. Xerostomia may be complicated by mouth sores, halitosis, and dental decay. Examination of the patient with xerostomia may reveal cracked lips, angular cheilitis, lack of salivary pooling, gingival inflammation, ulcers, and/or thrush. Multiple factors are associated with xerostomia in the palliative care patient, including decreased saliva secretion, dehydration, medications (e.g., anticholinergics), oxygen therapy, and mouth breathing. Once underlying conditions are addressed (if appropriate), xerostomia can be managed with basic mouth care, peppermint water, vitamin C, and artificial saliva substitutes.

107. C: Bone repair and formation is a balance between osteoblasts (bone-forming cells) and osteoclasts (bone-resorption cells). Bisphosphonates inhibit osteoclast activity, leading to decreased bone breakdown. The two primary therapeutic uses of bisphosphonate medication in the palliative care patient are treatment of hypercalcemia and bone pain. Patients with multiple myeloma or bony metastatic disease may experience improved pain management when bisphosphonate medications are added to the analgesic regimen. Typically, other analgesic therapy is also required for adequate pain control. Bisphosphonates also decrease the risk of pathological fracture and metastatic spinal cord compression in breast cancer and multiple myeloma patients with asymptomatic bone lesions.

108. B: Constipation is a common and unpleasant condition in the palliative care patient. Opioid-related bowel dysfunction is a common contributing factor, although constipation may also be secondary to intra-abdominal masses, other medications, electrolyte abnormalities (e.g., hypercalcemia), spinal cord compression, and poor oral intake. Constipation may cause Abdominal distension, abdominal pain, rectal pain, leakage of liquid stool, urinary retention, and agitation.

Pharmacologic management primarily consists of stool softeners and laxatives, which should be started with the initiation of opioid therapy in the palliative care patient. Nonpharmacologic measures (as tolerated) that help treat constipation include increased fluid and fiber intake, increased physical activity, and sitting upright for defecation attempts.

109. C: Seizures can be exhausting for patients and very upsetting for loved ones to witness. Management of acute seizure in the palliative care patient depends in part on the care setting and available routes for medication administration. Benzodiazepines are the medication of choice for treatment of acute seizures, and the oral or rectal route is preferred in the terminally ill patient, particularly in the home setting. Rectal diazepam is effective and easily administered. Although fosphenytoin and phenobarbital may be indicated for acute seizure treatment, they require intravenous or subcutaneous administration when used to treat ongoing seizure activity.

110. D: The primary risk factor for pressure injury development is immobility. Other contributing factors include decreased sensation (e.g., diabetic neuropathy), friction, shear, altered cognition, excessive skin moisture (e.g., incontinence), and advanced age. Most palliative care patients are at increased risk for pressure injury development due to progressive loss of mobility and impaired nutritional status as oral intake decreases.

111. D: Grief is defined as the emotional reaction to a significant loss. It is accompanied by a variety of manifestations: cognitive (e.g., impaired concentration, disbelief), emotional (e.g., sadness, anger, relief), and physical (e.g., appetite change, sleep disturbance, fatigue). Complicated grief is distinguished from uncomplicated grief primarily by duration, severity, and intensity of grief symptoms. Signs indicative of complicated grief (aside from duration of worsening symptoms beyond 6-12 months) include significant neglect of basic self-care, substance overuse/abuse, suicidality, and psychotic symptoms. Persistence of typical manifestations of grief two months after the death of a spouse is consistent with uncomplicated grief.

112. B: The signs and symptoms of impending death are often very similar, even between patients with very different terminal illnesses. The palliative care nurse should be familiar with the common signs and symptoms of impending death so that he or she can educate the patient and caregivers about the dying process. Each patient's goals for end-of-life care and the dying process should be honored as palliative care plans are formulated. Some patients may prefer to have only one or two loved ones present at the time of death, while others may prefer to be surrounded by many family members. Teaching caregivers the signs of impending death and ways to manage associated symptoms as they arise often results in decreased anxiety and fear about the dying process.

113. C: As with nausea and vomiting, opioid-associated sedation often improves several days after starting a particular medication. If intolerable sedative effects due to opioids continue, further management depends on whether the patient's pain is well controlled with the current opioid regimen. If the patient is pain-free (as in this case) and experiencing excessive opioid-related sedation, it is reasonable to attempt a dose reduction in the hope of maintaining effective pain management while reducing adverse effects. Other effective treatment strategies in the patient who does not tolerate a dose reduction include opioid switching at equianalgesic doses or addition of a psychostimulant medication. Use of prokinetic agents, such as metoclopramide, is not indicated or effective for the treatment of opioid-associated sedation.

114. B: Malignant ascites is most commonly associated with cancers of the breast, ovary, pancreas, and gastrointestinal tract. Ascites is difficult to prevent and can cause a great deal of suffering in the palliative care patient, including abdominal pain, bloating, shortness of breath, inability to lay flat, nausea, gastroesophageal reflux, and skin breakdown. Paracentesis consists of percutaneous drainage of up to 4-6 liters of ascitic fluid. This provides immediate relief to the patient, though ascites will gradually reaccumulate. Although invasive procedures are generally avoided in most palliative care patients with advanced malignancy, paracentesis for management of suffering due to malignant ascites is appropriate and effective. Although diuretics and oral fluid/sodium restriction may decrease ascites in some patients, those interventions take hours to days to improve symptoms.

115. C: This patient's symptoms (severe, intermittent suprapubic pain) are consistent with bladder spasms (detrusor muscle contractions). Bladder spasms may be caused by genitourinary inflammation (e.g., chemotherapy-related cystitis, radiation therapy), acute urinary tract infection, lower urinary tract obstruction (e.g., tumor), or indwelling catheter complications (e.g., occlusion, poor sizing). Treatment depends on the underlying cause. Excess caffeine or alcohol intake may exacerbate bladder spasms. Patients with bladder spasms are encouraged to drink plenty of fluids (if appropriate).

116. C: It is common for families to experience significant emotional stress as signs of impending death are developing, even if they have been well supported and educated about the final stages of a terminal illness. Family members often need compassionate, gentle reminders of the patient's preferences for end-of-life care and the futility of life-extending interventions as they relate to the patient's illness. Abandoning a family in this time of tremendous stress is inappropriate. It is important to assist families in continuing with the patient's plan of care without making them feel forced or bullied into a course of action. Preparation and support before death is impending make it much less likely that loved ones will abruptly attempt to change course as it becomes clear that death is imminent.

117. C: Significant limitations and challenges remain in the United States in the provision of high-quality end-of-life care across the full spectrum of patients and practice settings. The palliative care nurse is in an excellent position to advocate for improved end-of-life care legislation. Depending on the experience and comfort of the nurse, advocacy at the public policy level can consist of a wide variety of activities. Examples include becoming a member of professional organizations dedicated to advancing the cause of palliative care in the public arena, evaluating policy proposals, participating in the legislative process, engaging the media, building coalitions with other professional groups, and educating the public about palliative care issues. It is not appropriate for nurses to use their professional responsibilities to advance their own personal financial interests.

118. D: The essence of palliative care is the provision of holistic care to maximize quality of life in accordance with each patient's individual goals. Some patients may wish to maximize the duration of their life, while others may prioritize a specific task they want to accomplish before dying. The palliative care nurse should seek to elicit the patient's preferences, fears, and priorities with the goal of collaborating with the rest of the care team in developing a plan that best meets the patient's needs. In this case, the palliative care nurse can teach the patient and family strategies for managing symptoms when away from home, help arrange for portable supplies the patient may need (e.g., oxygen), identify resources the patient can access when traveling, etc. It is not appropriate for the nurse to discourage the patient or to tell the patient what his priorities should be.

119. B: As symptoms progress, patients and their caregivers need to be taught a variety of strategies for minimizing symptoms and maximizing patient comfort. Techniques for decreasing dyspnea include patient placement near a fan or open window, placement of the patient in the positions that decrease dyspnea (e.g., upright, leaning forward), oxygen administration, optimal timing and dosage of relevant medications, physical support during activities that increase breathlessness, and steady caregiver presence at the bedside (unless declined by the patient).

Breathlessness is an unpleasant and scary sensation for most patients; the presence of caregivers is an important factor in managing dyspnea.

120. A: Reflex urinary incontinence due to loss of neurological control of the detrusor muscle is characterized by unpredictable and often incomplete bladder emptying that is not accompanied by urgency or warning. Catheterization (either via intermittent catheterization or an indwelling urinary catheter) is usually required for management. Anticholinergic medications in conjunction with catheterization may also be helpful because of their inhibitory effect on bladder contractility. Pelvic floor muscle training is most useful in cases of stress incontinence. Antibiotics are helpful for cases of urinary incontinence caused by urinary tract infection. Fluid restriction is not appropriate for the treatment of urinary incontinence, although avoiding intake of large fluid volumes over a short period of time can be helpful.

121. B: Naloxone administration is rarely indicated in the palliative care patient because of the risk of extreme pain and possible autonomic crisis with rapid opioid reversal. With appropriate consideration of patient-related factors that may affect opioid metabolism and careful titration of opioid dosage, severe respiratory depression requiring naloxone administration should be rare in the palliative care setting. Alternative etiologies or contributing factors should be assessed in the palliative care patient with respiratory depression, such as other medications or impending death. Most patients exhibiting respiratory depression due to opioids will require only dose reduction and supportive care (e.g., stimulation, oxygen). Naloxone is indicated only for patients with significant respiratory depression (respiratory rate less than 8-10 breaths per minute) in association with marked reduction in level of consciousness and hypoxemia (oxygen saturation less than 90%). Naloxone should be administered in the minimum possible dose, with the goal of improving respiratory status while avoiding precipitation of a pain crisis or opioid withdrawal.

122. D: There are multiple analgesic medications, commonly referred to as "adjuvant" pain medications, that may be more effective than opioid medications at treating cancer pain. Adjuvant therapies for neuropathic pain include tricyclic antidepressants, anticonvulsants, steroids, local anesthetics, capsaicin, ketamine, and calcium channel blockers. Bisphosphonates are indicated for the treatment of bone pain (and hypercalcemia). Palliative ("terminal") sedation refers to the use of sedatives to treat pain or suffering in the palliative care patient when other treatment measures are ineffective. Increasing opioid doses to treat pain that is not opioid-responsive will not generally be effective.

123. C: Physiological pain assessment should include the patient's explanation of the pain's location, description (e.g., sharp, throbbing), intensity (e.g., 0-10 number scale), duration/timing, aggravating factors, alleviating factors, and any associated symptoms (e.g., shortness of breath). A thorough understanding of the physiological components of a patient's pain will make it easier to select an appropriate and effective analgesic agent/strategy. For example, a long-acting opioid is more effective for constant, dull pain than for sharp, intermittent incident pain. Although a complete pain assessment will include emotional, environmental, and cognitive factors affecting the patient's pain experience, those factors are distinct from the components of physiological pain assessment.

124. B: Gradually decreasing food and fluid intake is an expected event in the dying patient because of decreased nutritional need and declining interest in eating and drinking. The resulting dehydration may lead to increased patient comfort. Edema, respiratory difficulty, and skin discomfort may all improve with the dehydration that develops as the dying patient reduces oral intake. As the patient is less willing or able to swallow, other routes may be used for medication administration as needed (e.g., sublingual, rectal). Although it can be upsetting for family members when the dying patient is not able to eat or drink anymore, oral fluids should not be forced.

125. D: Pain is a subjective perception that has multiple contributing factors. Each patient's experience of pain will be unique. Two patients with physiologically identical injury or illness may experience a dramatically different degree of pain; therefore, it is not helpful to compare seemingly similar patients when it comes to pain assessment. Pain perception and reporting is affected by physiological, emotional, behavioral, cultural, and environmental factors.

126. C: Analgesic medication choice should take into account a variety of factors. These include pain severity, type, and duration, in addition to available routes of administration and underlying medical issues that may affect drug metabolism or adverse effects. In general, the initial treatment of mild pain in the palliative care patient should consist of nonopioid medications, in addition to nonpharmacologic pain management strategies. Medications that would be appropriate for initial treatment of mild pain are acetaminophen and/or NSAIDs, such as ibuprofen.

127. C: Maintaining important family rituals and traditions, even if they need to be changed somewhat to accommodate a patient's illness, is important for enhancing the well-being of both patients and their family caregivers. Life-threatening illness inevitably disrupts daily routines, but it can be very therapeutic when traditions are honored even in the midst of serious illness. The process of "redefining" involves making adjustments in tasks and routines that the patient is no longer able to engage in because of disease progression. Important nursing interventions for this patient's caregivers include encouraging them to express their feelings about what has changed, reminding them of what remains possible, and assisting them in finding new ways to engage in the activities that are most meaningful for them.

128. A: Breaking bad news about disease progression or prognosis is an extremely important skill for all palliative care providers to develop. Patients have the right to make independent, well-informed choices about treatment, life, and death. This depends on having access to complete information, even information that is difficult to hear or accept. It should not be up to the provider what information the patient receives. However, if a patient requests that certain details be withheld or communicated to an alternative loved one, that should be honored. Common barriers to effective communication in any clinical discussion include a language barrier, overuse of complex medical terminology, provider discomfort, and failure to establish a setting in which there is adequate time and space for emotional responses and follow-up questions. It is often very helpful for patients to have supportive loved ones present for conversations about prognosis and progression.

129. B: The transition into palliative care can be scary and difficult for patients and families. There is a great deal of uncertainty when a patient leaves the inpatient setting and changes care teams, and still has symptoms related to ongoing illness. The palliative care nurse is in an excellent position to help patients make that transition. The hospice team should, ideally, be included in formulating the plan of care prior to discharge. The nurse can help ensure that necessary equipment and medications are available without interruption to minimize the risk of poorly controlled symptoms (e.g., pain). Any necessary education to help patients and caregivers make it through the first days at home should be completed before discharge, and patients should know how to quickly access additional support if unexpected challenges arise. Certification of initial hospice eligibility must be performed by a physician.

130. C: Multidimensional and well-supported programs designed to support palliative care nurses are crucial given the increased potential for occupational stress and burnout brought on by the psychosocial challenges inherent in palliative care. Important components of a supportive framework include opportunities for community-building among providers, emphasis on self-care activities, education about the signs of occupational stress, and ongoing opportunities to check in and improve upon existing support programs. Lack of attention to one's own physical, emotional, and spiritual needs will make it impossible for the palliative care nurse to provide competent and compassionate care to patients.

131. A: Many patients will explore alternative and complementary therapies to treat symptoms of their primary disease or adverse effects associated with treatment. Most of these therapies emphasize the whole patient, the body's capacity to heal from within, and the mind-body connection. Examples include yoga, hypnosis, guided imagery, acupuncture, massage, aromatherapy, art/music therapy, and Reiki. Studies have shown that some cancer patients experience decreased pain, anxiety, depression, and fatigue after receiving massage therapy. The palliative care nurse should be familiar with the basic principles of alternative therapies, as well as possible complications. Massage therapy is discouraged in the patient with a bleeding propensity, over bones with known metastatic lesions, over known vessel thromboses, and over surgical sites or skin rashes. There is no evidence to suggest that massage therapy will decrease the effectiveness of oral pain medications. In the absence of concern for dangerous interactions or effects of complementary therapies, palliative care patients should not be discouraged from exploring alternative therapy for symptom relief.

132. D: It is important for the palliative care nurse to understand the difference between physical dependence, tolerance, and addiction to pain medications. One of the remaining barriers to adequate pain control in the palliative care patient is patient and/or provider concern for the development of addiction to pain medications. Physical dependence occurs when the body has adapted to long-term use of a medication so that rapid dose reduction or discontinuation of the medication produces symptoms of withdrawal. Tolerance occurs when the body adjusts to a stable medication dose, resulting in a need for increased dosage of the medication to achieve the same effect. Patients who are experiencing end-of-dose failure have breakthrough pain or increase in pain because their medication is not lasting long enough. This is commonly referred to as "clock-watching" and is often mistaken for drug-seeking behavior due to addiction. Psychological dependence (i.e., addiction) is characterized by a lack of control over medication use, compulsive medication use, and continued use despite harmful physiological or social effects.

133. C: Spontaneous (or idiopathic) pain occurs spontaneously without a predictable inciting factor. Incident pain arises fairly predictably in association with a certain inciting event, such as movement or wound irrigation. Pain associated with end-of-dose failure arises as the time for the next scheduled dose of analgesic medication approaches. Pain due to end-of-dose failure may be misinterpreted as drug-seeking behavior, particularly if a patient is becoming tolerant to a particular analgesic agent.

134. B: The palliative care nurse is in a unique position with hospice patients and should embrace his or her role as an important patient advocate when ethical conflicts and challenges arise. Far from being a peripheral care provider, the palliative care nurse is an excellent liaison between the patient and the rest of the palliative care team. The nurse is familiar with patient's end-of-life goals, psychosocial strengths and challenges, functional status, and ongoing medical and psychological needs. The nurse is an important advocate for the patient, especially in more clinical settings where the patient may feel intimidated or be unable to express preferences. The nurse can help the entire team identify and work through the issues that lead to ethical conflicts.

135. B: Patients and families dealing with progressive cognitive and/or neuromuscular disease benefit greatly from palliative care services. Although each patient's clinical and psychosocial course is unique, these nonmalignant neurological conditions generally progress along a predictable path toward disability and, ultimately, death. In contrast, multiple sclerosis in most patients is initially of the relapsing-remitting variant; in other words, the sporadic neurological symptoms a patient is experiencing spontaneously resolve without any residual sequelae. Many of these patients go on to develop progressive neurological decline later in the course of the disease. Huntington's disease is a progressive, inherited disease marked by psychiatric symptoms, involuntary movements, and cognitive decline. Alzheimer's disease leads to progressive decline in cognition and memory and is marked by specific neuropathological findings in the brain. Amyotrophic lateral sclerosis (ALS) is a neuromuscular disease that primarily results in progressive muscular weakness.

136. A: The National Consensus Project's Clinical Practice Guidelines for Quality Palliative Care were designed to improve the quality of palliative care delivery across all age groups and practice settings. The practice guidelines are a resource for palliative care providers as well as a "comprehensive description of what constitutes a high-quality palliative care clinical service." The Practice Guidelines are divided into eight domains: structure and processes of care, physical aspects of care, psychological and psychiatric aspects of care, social aspects of care, spiritual/religious/existential aspects of care, cultural aspects of care, care of the imminently dying patient, and ethical and legal aspects of care.

137. A: Congestive heart failure causes a variety of symptoms that can greatly reduce a palliative care patient's quality of life. Pain is a common symptom, especially chest pain due to myocardial ischemia and extremity pain due to edema and arthritis. Dyspnea is also common in the patient with terminal heart failure, primarily due to pulmonary edema that develops as a result of cardiac pump failure. Other common symptoms include fatigue, depression, sleeping difficulties, and poor appetite. Opioid pain medications are indicated and effective for both pain and dyspnea in these patients. As the patient transitions to palliative care, the entire treatment regimen (including diet, medications, and implanted cardiac devices) should be evaluated. The patient's goals for symptom management and end-of-life care should dictate the specifics of the treatment plan.

138. D: The American Nurses Association's position on pain management in end-of-life care is clear: The palliative care nurse is both ethically justified and professionally obligated to administer the analgesic dosage required to sufficiently manage the patient's pain, even if concern exists over hastening death. A 1997 Supreme Court case upheld this principle. Because of opioid tolerance, there is no established maximum dosage for opioid medication. Placebo administration is not ethically justified in palliative care patients without their consent (e.g., as part of a double-blind research study) and is definitely not indicated in the setting of inadequate pain control.

139. B: Most metastatic disease to the bone arises in association with cancers of the breast, prostate, thyroid, lung, and kidney. The most common presenting symptom of bony metastasis is localized, progressive pain at the site of the metastatic lesion. Bony metastasis may also present with pathological fracture due to bony destruction at the site of the metastatic lesion. Pain or pathological fracture due to metastatic bone disease may be a patient's first symptom of the primary malignancy. Although extensive bone metastases may cause hypercalcemia, this would be an unusual presenting symptom.

140. B: Providing compassionate end-of-life care is the cornerstone of palliative care, and the relationship at the core of palliative care is between the nurse and the patient. An authentic, caring relationship between the palliative care nurse and patient will greatly enhance the patient's end-of-life experience and will also provide great satisfaction to the nurse. Although efficient care and evidence-based care are important in all medical settings, the patient's care will be suboptimal in the absence of a meaningful relationship between nurse and patient.

141. C: Palliative care patients commonly have multiple factors that lead to increased risk for aspiration events. Altered mental status—due to medication effect, stroke, or brain mass—leads to decreased airway protective reflexes. Impaired swallowing coordination (dysphagia) may be due to a variety of factors, including respiratory disease, advanced age, general debility, critical illness, and neurological/neuromuscular disease, such as Parkinson's disease or amyotrophic lateral sclerosis. Aspiration may occur during a clearly identifiable event, or may be "silent" without a definitive choking event.

142. A: Under the Medicare Hospice Benefit, the hospice services available to a patient who resides in a nursing home are no different than the services available to a patient living at home. However, hospice care remains underused in nursing home patients because of a variety of factors, including difficulty predicting life expectancy for patients with nonmalignant disease and lack of effective collaboration between nursing home and hospice care agencies. A nursing home patient receiving hospice care has a plan of care developed and implemented by the hospice care team, including symptom management, psychosocial support, and provision of medical supplies. Hospice care is provided primarily by the hospice care team. Ideally, collaboration and communication between hospice team members and nursing home staff allows for shared assessment and care responsibilities in a manner that best serves the patient's needs.

143. D: Elderly patients in all settings are at a markedly increased risk for accidental falls. Underlying medical and age-related conditions create increased risk of falls, which leads to increased risk of medical complications. Morbidity and mortality rates are significantly increased for elderly patients in the months after an accidental fall. Predisposing factors that contribute to falls in the elderly population include underlying acute illness (e.g., infection), chronic medical conditions that may impair balance or strength (e.g., arthritis, orthostatic hypotension, cancer), medication effects, and environmental hazards (e.g., stairs, inadequate lighting). Identifying patients at increased risk for falls, and modifying contributing risk factors, can greatly decrease a patient's likelihood of accidental falls.

144. C: The essential goals of palliative care are the relief of pain and suffering (physical, spiritual, and psychosocial) in the terminally ill patient, optimizing quality of life in the time remaining, and supporting the patient and loved ones through the dying process. Meeting all these goals requires a team made up of a variety of professionals (e.g., physician, nurse, social worker, pharmacist, pastoral care) in addition to the patient and family members. To continue to meet the patient's needs as illness progresses, the most effective model includes all team members meeting on a regular basis to elicit the patient's goals and preferences regarding end-of-life care, identify challenges and possible solutions, and formulate the care plan that best meets the patient's needs. As illness progresses, the patient's goals and needs may change, making ongoing team meetings crucial for ensuring that the plan continues to meet the patient's needs.

145. B: It is common for patients to require transfer among various palliative care settings as illness progresses or family availability/resources change. Open lines of communication and collaboration between care providers in multiple disciplines is critical for maintaining uninterrupted, high-quality palliative care as patients transfer between care settings. Providers in each setting should make it a priority to be aware of other palliative care resources in the community and to be familiar with the strengths and weaknesses of each as they pertain to specific patient situations. Ideally, when transfer occurs from one setting to another or from one set of providers to another, there is open and repeated communication between teams both before and after the transfer of care.

146. A: Palliative care nursing is a career with the potential for significant job-related stress. The usual issues contributing to nurses' stress (e.g., workload, shift, hierarchical challenges) are compounded by grief for patient deaths and by ethical quandaries that may arise with end-of-life care. As with all careers, a large determinant of long-term job satisfaction is the extent to which the nurse's overall well-being is enhanced by the work. Emphasis on skills, compensation, or career advancement does not provide the same degree of personal fulfillment as a deeply meaningful and personal connection to both the patients and the core values of palliative care nursing.

147. A: Patients (and families, when appropriate) should be the centerpiece of interdisciplinary palliative care team discussions. The essence of palliative care is to provide end-of-life care that is formulated around each patient's individual goals and preferences. Even if the patient is not willing or able to participate, the patient's wishes (to the maximal extent they can be determined) should be the primary determinant driving the discussion. Patients may need to be reminded that they are the experts when it comes to the symptoms they are experiencing, as well as their goals, values, preferences, fears, and needs. The expertise of the rest of the team is applied to addressing those things. Although designation of a healthcare power of attorney should be encouraged, it is important for patients to remember that they retain full power to make decisions unless and until they are no longer able to do so.

148. C: The hospice home health aide or certified nursing assistant (CNA) is a valuable member of the hospice care team. Often, the hospice home health aide is at the patient's bedside more than any other member of the care team, aside from family members. Home health aides assist with hygiene and toileting/continence, activities of daily living, patient transfer, light housekeeping, and patient/family support. Some home health aides may also assist with medication administration. Home health aides are supervised by the hospice nurse and carry out the plan of care as instructed by the hospice nurse. While the home health aide is an important source of information about changes in the patient's status, he or she should not provide medical advice or professional nursing care.

149. B: Pain is a multifactorial and highly subjective experience, making comprehensive pain assessment crucial in the palliative care patient. Assessment of the physiological/sensory components of pain (e.g., location, intensity, quality) is often the focus of pain assessment. Other contributing factors to a patient's experience of pain should be evaluated and addressed as well. Sociocultural aspects of pain that should be assessed include preexisting cultural or religious beliefs about pain, as well as the impact of the patient's pain on the patient's role in his or her family, occupation, and cultural community. Affective or psychological components of pain include the patient's emotional experience with and response to pain. Preexisting anxiety, depression, or loss of hope will often significantly impact a patient's response to physical pain. Conversely, poorly controlled physical pain may harm a patient's mood and ability to cope.

150. B: Radiation therapy may be used primarily for curative purposes, in combination with other cancer therapies, or for palliation of cancer-related symptoms. Adverse effects are common and include nausea, fatigue, mucosal irritation of mucous membranes in the radiation field, hair loss, and skin changes. Typically, dermatologic adverse effects of radiation are observed 2-3 weeks after the initiation of therapy. Skin reactions include dryness, flaking, itching, redness, hyperpigmentation, oozing, and crusting. Skin care for radiation-associated skin changes includes loose-fitting clothes, avoidance of irritants (e.g., lotion, deodorant), use of topical steroids, and protection from sun exposure.

Practice Test #2

1. A bedbound patient has a 1.5-inch foam overlay over her mattress. The nurse places her hand under the overlay and finds that the overlay has compressed to 0.75 inches. This indicates:

a. Bottoming out
b. Adequate support
c. Excess wear
d. Moisture retention

2. Which of the following drugs used for terminal sedation is a very rapid, short-acting benzodiazepine?

a. Pentobarbital
b. Propofol
c. Midazolam
d. Lorazepam

3. In the last stages of amyotrophic lateral sclerosis (ALS), almost all patients:

a. Exhibit signs of dementia.
b. Require mechanical ventilation to breathe.
c. Have weight gain.
d. Exhibit slight slurring of speech.

4. The most effective treatment for relief of an elevated temperature of 38.8° C (102° F) is:

a. Acetaminophen or ibuprofen
b. Aspirin
c. Alcohol bath
d. Cold bath

5. A palliative care patient undergoing chemotherapy has developed myelosuppression. The patient should be advised to avoid all of the following EXCEPT:

a. Strenuous activities
b. Alcohol
c. Shaving the legs, underarms, or face
d. High-protein diet

6. A patient with ovarian cancer uses fentanyl patches to control pain. She complains that she suddenly has difficulty urinating and only dribbles small amounts. Her bladder is not distended, but the patient complains of bilateral pain in the flank areas. She has no fever. Her electrolyte count shows slight hyperkalemia. The most likely cause is:

a. Upper urinary tract obstruction
b. Bladder neck obstruction
c. Bladder infection
d. Opioid-induced deficiency of detrusor muscle contraction

7. A hospice patient develops a severe and spreading infection of a draining pressure injury, resulting in markedly increased pain and fever. Culture shows a methicillin-resistant *Staphylococcus aureus* (MRSA) infection. The best treatment is:

a. Addition of adjuvant pain medications to current pain management
b. Antibiotics and modification in pain management
c. Increased opioid dose
d. Contact precautions

8. When the hospice nurse arrives at the home of a patient whose death is imminent, the daughter states, "I can't stay in the room when Dad dies! I can't stand the thought!" The best response is:

a. "You will regret it if you don't."
b. "Your father would want you with him."
c. "I'll stay with him and you can come and go as you feel comfortable."
d. "Is there someone else who can stay with him?"

9. When the nurse visits a hospice patient at home, he states, "I can't stand this pain anymore. I should just shoot myself and be done with it." The best initial response is:

a. "I understand why you feel that way. I'll ask the doctor to prescribe an antidepressant for you."
b. "I'm sure you don't really mean that."
c. "Let's work together to find better ways to manage your pain."
d. "Do you have a plan to hurt yourself?"

10. A hospice patient with prostate cancer has recently completed a course of radiation to relieve spinal compression from bone metastasis. His pain is well controlled with fentanyl, but he is fearful and has developed tremors and jerking movements of his extremities that are keeping him awake at night. The most likely cause is:

a. Brain metastasis
b. Spinal damage
c. Anxiety
d. Opioid-induced myoclonus

11. A patient reports having a brief episode of syncope during which she almost blacked out. When evaluating this patient, which of the following is the most important information initially?

a. Duration of the episode
b. Activity immediately prior to the episode
c. Symptoms following the episode
d. List of medications

12. A patient has experienced rapid gastrointestinal bleeding. Which of the following is most effective in the initial evaluation of the extent of anemia?

a. Hemoglobin
b. Hematocrit
c. Clinical signs
d. Arterial PO_2

13. A palliative care patient has a severe infection and sepsis, and has subsequently developed bleeding from her venous puncture site, gastric distention, petechiae, purpura, and severe hypotension. Both her prothrombin and partial thromboplastin times are increased, while platelet count and fibrinogen are decreased. Red blood cells are fragmented. The most likely diagnosis is:

a. Disseminated intravascular coagulation (DIC)
b. Multiple organ dysfunction syndrome
c. Aplastic anemia
d. Hypovolemic anemia

14. A patient with lung cancer suddenly complains of acute pleuritic pain on the left side. He exhibits dyspnea, tachypnea, tachycardia, and slight cough. Auscultation shows decreased breath sounds on the left. The most likely diagnosis is:

a. Atelectasis
b. Pneumothorax
c. Pneumonia
d. Cardiac tamponade

15. Which of the following exercises is best for chronic obstructive pulmonary disease (COPD) patients to promote effective expulsion of trapped air from the lungs?

a. Inspiratory muscle training
b. Pursed-lip breathing
c. Paced walking
d. Diaphragmatic breathing

16. Which of the following heart sounds is an indication of heart failure in an older adult?

a. Opening snap
b. Ejection click
c. Friction rub
d. S3

17. Chronic renal failure is characterized by all of the following EXCEPT:

a. Hypokalemia
b. Sodium and fluid retention
c. Anemia
d. Metabolic acidosis

18. A hospice patient has suffered a stroke in the left hemisphere, causing right-sided paralysis. Which of the following symptoms should the nurse anticipate?

a. Aphasia
b. Nausea and vomiting
c. Respiratory and cardiac dysfunction
d. Left-sided neglect

19. A palliative care patient has been drinking heavily and smoking. He states that he has been having severe episodes of chest pain at about the same time each afternoon when he is watching television. Which diagnosis is most likely?

a. Esophageal varices
b. Stable angina
c. Unstable angina
d. Variant (Prinzmetal) angina

20. The most common type of pathological fracture found in patients in palliative care is:

a. Spinal fracture
b. Femur fracture
c. Wrist fracture
d. Ankle fracture

21. Which of the following drugs is most likely to cause extrapyramidal symptoms, such as akinesia and dystonia?

a. Phenytoin
b. Hydromorphone
c. Haloperidol
d. Fluoxetine

22. When treating anxiety in a geriatric patient, which type of medication is preferred?

a. Short-acting benzodiazepine
b. Long-acting benzodiazepine
c. Tricyclic antidepressant
d. β-adrenergic agent

23. A palliative care patient requires intravenous therapy for about 6-8 weeks. Which of the following central venous access devices is most commonly used for this duration?

a. Non-tunneled central catheter
b. Peripherally inserted central catheter (PICC)
c. Tunneled central catheter
d. Implantable port

24. Opioid tolerance is characterized by all of the following EXCEPT:

a. The patient experiences markedly increased side effects.
b. The patient complains of pain much more severe than expected with the condition.
c. The patient needs excessively high doses to control pain.
d. The patient experiences very few side effects (such as drowsiness).

25. The complementary therapy that is probably the most effective adjunct therapy for pain is:

a. Music therapy
b. Therapeutic touch
c. Massage
d. Acupuncture

26. Nonsteroidal anti-inflammatory drugs (NSAIDs) are contraindicated as co-adjuvants due to increased bleeding risks with which of the following?

a. Anticonvulsants
b. Corticosteroids
c. Bisphosphonates
d. Antidepressants

27. Withholding food and fluids in the dying patient can cause increased ketone production and electrolyte imbalance that result in:

a. Decreased pain and discomfort
b. Increased respiratory distress
c. Nausea and vomiting
d. Increased peripheral edema

28. An elderly male with a history of enlarged prostate is receiving hydromorphone for pain as well as a tricyclic antidepressant. He is most at risk for the adverse effect of:

a. Myoclonus
b. Pruritus
c. Urinary retention
d. Delirium

29. Which adjuvant drug is most appropriate for osteolytic bone pain?

a. Tricyclic antidepressants
b. Anticonvulsants
c. Corticosteroids
d. Bisphosphonates

30. As a patient nears death, his wife begins to imitate some of his behaviors. Which type of grief response does this represent?

a. Physical
b. Spiritual
c. Sociocultural
d. Psychological

31. A dying patient has taken no fluids for 24 hours. Which measure is most appropriate to alleviate discomfort from dehydration?

a. Providing mouth care and moistening mucous membranes
b. Administering intravenous fluids
c. Placing ice chips in the patient's mouth
d. Encouraging sips of fluid

32. All of the following are the direct result of decreased cardiac output and intravascular volume in the dying patient EXCEPT:

a. Hypotension
b. Bradycardia
c. Mottling
d. Peripheral and/or central cyanosis

33. When evaluating a patient for pain management, the initial objective is to:

a. Identify treatable causes of the pain.
b. Assess the level of pain.
c. Choose an effective pain medication.
d. Assess the patient's psychological status.

34. A patient with advanced prostate cancer has been treated with diethylstilbestrol (DES). A common adverse effect is:

a. Hot flashes
b. Increased libido
c. Gynecomastia
d. Bone pain

35. A patient with gastric distention has developed recurring hiccups. Which of the following medical treatments is most indicated?

a. Haloperidol
b. Baclofen or chlorpromazine
c. Metoclopramide
d. Omeprazole

36. Palliative care can begin when:

a. A patient is diagnosed with a life-threatening disease.
b. A patient's life expectancy is less than one year.
c. A patient's life expectancy is 6 months or less.
d. A patient requests palliative care.

37. An opioid-naive patient is one who:

a. Is not responding to opioids
b. Is resistant to opioids
c. Has been taking daily opioids routinely
d. Has not been taking daily opioids routinely

38. A patient is nearing death and has started to develop a pressure injury on the sacral area but moans loudly and is resistive when the nurses try to turn him. The best action is to:

a. Turn the patient frequently to prevent further skin deterioration.
b. Allow the patient to lie undisturbed as much as possible.
c. Increase pain medication so that the patient can be turned.
d. Transfer the patient to a bed with an alternating pressure mattress.

39. A hospice patient with a coccygeal pressure injury has a Foley catheter (18 Fr/30 cc) for incontinence but develops bladder spasms about 4 weeks after the catheter is inserted. All of the following are appropriate to reduce the bladder spasms EXCEPT:

a. Remove the catheter and provide disposable underwear.
b. Provide anticholinergic medications, such as oxybutynin.
c. Change the catheter.
d. Insert a Foley catheter of a smaller size or with a smaller balloon.

40. According to the American Nurses Association (ANA) Code of Ethics for Nurses, nurses must support a patient's autonomy and self-determination. If a 44-year-old Asian female patient has stated a treatment preference but plans to leave the ultimate decision to family members, the nurse should:

a. Try to convince the patient to assert herself.
b. Recognize that cultural values regarding individualism vary, and respect the patient's right to be guided by her family.
c. Tell the family that the patient should be the one to make the decision.
d. Ask the ethics committee to intervene.

41. A daughter returns home to assist her parents when her mother becomes terminally ill, but the father disagrees with the mother's choices regarding terminal care. The daughter sides with her father, and they apply pressure on the mother to change her mind. Under Bowen family systems theory, this is an example of:

a. Triangle theory
b. Projection
c. Transmission
d. Emotional isolation

42. All of the following communication skills are essential for collaboration EXCEPT:

a. Ability to make casual conversation
b. Competent public speaking ability
c. Competent writing skills
d. Unassertive approach

43. Which of the following is most effective for including the patient or family in the development of the interdisciplinary plan of care?

a. "Please ask us if you have any questions."
b. "We will keep you informed of all plans."
c. "What would you like to include in your plan of care?"
d. "How do you feel about your plan of care?"

44. The National Consensus Project's Domains of Quality Palliative Care include all of the following EXCEPT:

a. Physical aspects of care
b. Economic aspects of care
c. Cultural aspects of care
d. Psychological and psychiatric aspects of care

45. A debilitated patient has developed chronic constipation with opioid use. Which of the following is recommended to prevent or treat constipation?

a. Reduce the dose of the opioid.
b. Administer bulking agents (such as psyllium).
c. Force fluids.
d. Administer a stool laxative or softener.

46. Two staff nurses in the hospice unit disagree about the best way to carry out duties, resulting in ongoing conflict and their refusal to work together. The first step in resolving this conflict is to:

a. Allow both individuals to present their side of the conflict without bias.
b. Encourage them to reach a compromise.
c. Tell them they are violating professional standards of conduct.
d. Make a decision about the matter.

47. For disposal of used needles and lancets in the home, all of the following are acceptable EXCEPT:

a. A commercially purchased hard plastic sharps container
b. A clear glass jar with metal lid
c. A hard plastic opaque bleach bottle
d. A secure metal container

48. The nurse is in the room and attending the immediate and extended family of a dying infant during the death vigil. The mother is very upset and angry with the doctor for not saving her child. The most appropriate action for the nurse is to:

a. Reassure the family that the child's suffering will soon be over.
b. Sit quietly, and interact with the family if they desire.
c. Explain to the mother that the doctor is not to blame.
d. Hug the mother to provide comfort.

49. The nurse is teaching a patient to manage his pain pump for patient-controlled analgesia (PCA). Although the nurse explains at least three times, the patient asks the same questions over and over. The nurse provides a pamphlet with illustrations, but the patient barely looks at them and says he can't figure out what he needs to do. The best approach is probably to:

a. Suggest a different method of pain control.
b. Arrange for someone else to manage the equipment.
c. Allow a rest period, and then start again with instructions.
d. Allow the patient to practice with actual equipment.

50. Traditionally, all of the following are part of Islamic burial rituals EXCEPT:

a. Bathing the body
b. Cremating the body
c. Placing a shroud around the body
d. Reciting a funeral prayer

51. A common respiratory pattern found in dying patients is:

a. Cheyne-Stokes respirations
b. Kussmaul respirations
c. Tachypnea
d. Bradypnea

52. A cancer patient has developed white lesions on the tongue and inside of the cheeks. The tissue is irritated and painful and is bleeding slightly. Which treatment is indicated?

a. An antibiotic, such as tetracycline
b. Artificial saliva, such as Salivart
c. Antifungal medication, such a nystatin oral suspension
d. Mucous moisturizer, such as lemon-glycerin swabs

53. Acetaminophen is contraindicated as an adjuvant drug for patients with:

a. Intense pain
b. Gastrointestinal bleeding
c. Neurological disorders
d. Liver disease

54. A patient is dying of multiple sclerosis. Which of the following statements by a caregiver most indicates a risk for patient abuse?

a. "There's no reason for Mother to be incontinent! The next time, she can just lie in it!"
b. "Sometimes I just wish Mother would die and get it over with."
c. "I'm so tired of getting up at night. Sometimes I feel like crying."
d. "I don't know how much longer I can do this without help."

55. For the hospice nurse, all of the following are part of formal closure activities after a patient dies EXCEPT:

a. Visiting the family
b. Sending a card of condolence
c. Helping the family make funeral arrangements
d. Telephoning family members

56. For quality/performance improvement, the best tool to determine methods to streamline processes is:

a. Root-cause analysis
b. Tracer methodology
c. Family survey
d. Staff survey

57. A dying patient is experiencing severe breathlessness and is gasping for breath. The patient is opioid-tolerant and is taking parenteral morphine to control pain. Which of the following is likely to be most effective to relieve the discomfort associated with dyspnea?

a. Increase morphine dose by 2.5 mg.
b. Provide the patient with oxygen.
c. Add 5 mg of morphine orally every 4 hours.
d. Position the patient with the head of the bed elevated.

58. A Hmong patient with stage IV ovarian cancer is dying but tells the nurse that a Hmong shaman is coming to provide a healing, which she believes may cure her. The best response for the nurse to give is:

a. "That is not realistic in your condition."
b. "If you believe, then a cure is possible."
c. "You will need your doctor's permission."
d. "What can I do to help?"

59. The primary criterion for referral to a hospice program is:

a. Severe intractable pain
b. Life-threatening disease
c. Probability that death will occur within 6 months
d. Do not resuscitate (DNR) order

60. A dying patient has bladder incontinence and her skin is becoming irritated. She is increasingly confused and somnolent but asks for water. Turning is painful to her. The best solution is:

a. Disposable underwear
b. Skin barriers
c. Withholding fluids
d. Foley catheter for urinary drainage

61. According to the National Center for Complementary and Alternative Medicine, which of the following is an example of a whole medical system?

a. Acupuncture
b. Meditation
c. Vitamin therapy
d. Massage

62. When preparing written materials for patients, what readability level would be appropriate for a homogeneous adult patient group in an affluent area?

a. Grade 6 level
b. Grade 9 level
c. Grade 3 level
d. Grade 12 level

63. Which of the following is a violation of professional boundaries on the part of the nurse?

a. The nurse accepts a box of chocolates from a patient's daughter to be shared by all unit staff.
b. The nurse confides to the patient that he, like the patient, is getting a divorce, so he understands the patient's stress.
c. The nurse assists a patient in placing a call to his landlord so the patient can explain that he cannot pay the rent on time.
d. The nurse finds a patient crying and places his hand on the patient's shoulder.

64. A hospice patient with congestive heart failure has developed dependent edema of the lower extremities. All of the following are appropriate treatments EXCEPT:

a. Elevate legs.
b. Apply graded elastic compression stockings.
c. Administer diuretics.
d. Advise bed rest.

65. Self-determined life closure is indicated by:

a. Completion of advance directives
b. Death in the home rather than in a hospital
c. Request for a "do not resuscitate" (DNR) order
d. Honoring the patient's wishes regarding end-of-life care

66. The interdisciplinary team is considering adding a member to help coordinate care for an increasing number of pediatric patients. The most appropriate addition would be:

a. A child life specialist
b. An occupational therapist
c. A dietitian
d. A play therapist

67. A 76-year-old female with end-stage heart failure was referred for hospice care by her physician 6 months earlier (two 90-day periods), but she is still alive. A staff nurse asks the certified hospice and palliative nurse if the patient will be removed from hospice care. The best response is:

a. "She will be removed from hospice care until her condition worsens because she has exceeded the 6-month period."
b. "She has exhausted all of her hospice care benefits and will be removed from hospice care."
c. "She can continue with hospice care as long as the physician authorizes the care every 60 days."
d. "She can continue with hospice care if the physician continues to authorize care every 90 days."

68. Which of the following should require input from all members of the interdisciplinary team?

a. Titrating pain medications
b. Developing the plan of care
c. Instructing the patient in stress reduction techniques
d. Managing skin care

69. A family member stops the nurse and asks, "Could you tell me what is wrong with the patient across the hall from my father? He seems so agitated." The response that complies with the Health Insurance Portability and Accountability Act (HIPAA) is:

a. "The law doesn't allow me to give out any information about patients in order to protect their privacy and safety."
b. "His daughter is in the lounge. You can go ask her."
c. "Why are you asking?"
d. "He has cancer, like your father."

70. A patient with cognitive impairment has pancreatic cancer. Nonverbal behavior that can indicate pain includes all of the following EXCEPT:

a. Rapid, labored breathing
b. Moaning
c. Grimacing
d. Excessive sleeping

71. A patient's son insists that he should make all decisions regarding patient care even though the patient is alert and able to make decisions. The best approach is to:

a. Inform the son that the patient has the legal right to make the decisions.
b. Inform the patient that the son insists on making decisions for the patient.
c. Refer the issue to the ethics committee.
d. Arrange a family meeting with the patient, the son, and healthcare providers to discuss the patient's wishes.

72. When evaluating outcomes data for evidence-based practice, the type of data that includes measures of mortality, longevity, and cost-effectiveness is:

a. Clinical
b. Psychosocial
c. Integrative
d. Physiological

73. A patient has been receiving parenteral morphine sulfate at a dose of 10 mg every 4 hours but will be switched to an oral equianalgesic. All of the following are acceptable choices EXCEPT:

a. Codeine, 180 mg every 4 hours
b. Oxycodone controlled-release, 40 mg every 12 hours
c. Hydrocodone, 30 mg every 4 hours
d. Morphine controlled-release, 90 mg every 12 hours

74. When assessing a patient with dysarthria, the best approach is to:

a. Speak loudly and clearly.
b. Ask yes/no questions.
c. Ask questions requiring a summary of information.
d. Use visual aids to communicate ideas to the patient.

75. A rescue dose should be what percentage of the hourly parenteral opioid dose?

a. 5-15%
b. 10-20%
c. 25-50%
d. 50-70%

76. When the nurse delegates a task to another healthcare provider, the most important consideration when choosing the right person is:

a. Availability
b. Reliability
c. Education/skills
d. Years of experience

77. A dying patient with lung cancer develops sudden onset of confusion, restlessness, and anxiety and begins to moan, grimace, and thrash about the bed. The most likely cause is:

a. Increased pain
b. Terminal delirium
c. Brain metastasis
d. Stroke

78. Disadvantages of providing intravenous (IV) fluids for hydration to the terminally ill patient include all of the following EXCEPT:

a. It may hasten death.
b. It may increase urinary output and incontinence.
c. It may result in congestive heart failure.
d. It may result in skin breakdown.

79. Which is the most critical skill for a nurse collaborating in an interdisciplinary team?

a. Patience
b. Assertiveness
c. Empathy with others
d. Willingness to compromise

80. Signs of death can include all of the following EXCEPT:

a. Incontinence of urine and/or feces
b. Pinpoint pupils
c. Waxy pallor
d. Lack of heartbeat and respirations

81. A patient with pancreatic cancer (stage IV) is requiring increasing doses of an opioid to control the pain. The most likely reason is:

a. Progression of the disease
b. Addiction
c. Tolerance
d. Dependence

82. A bedridden patient with advanced liver cancer has had right abdominal pain but is now complaining of pain in the right shoulder. The most likely cause is:

a. Improper positioning
b. Bony metastasis
c. Referred pain
d. Pulled muscle

83. Which of the following tests is most accurate for determining acute changes in nutritional status to monitor dietary status for a patient with cachexia?

a. Transferrin
b. Total protein
c. Albumin
d. Prealbumin

84. A dying patient suddenly worsens, and death appears imminent within a few hours. It is 2 a.m. Exhausted family members went home at midnight to sleep, expecting the patient to survive the night. The nurse should:

a. Wait until 7 a.m. to call the family so they can rest.
b. Contact the family immediately so they can return.
c. Wait until after the patient dies to contact the family.
d. Observe the patient frequently and call the family when the patient is nearer death.

85. The most important criterion for determining the degree of a patient's pain is:

a. Physical indications, such as grimacing or guarding
b. Moaning
c. Patient report
d. Patient history

86. A dying patient is cared for in the home by her daughter, who states that no one else in her family understands how exhausting cooking, cleaning, and caregiving can be. The most appropriate referral is to a:

a. Caregiver support group
b. Psychologist
c. Meals-on-wheels program
d. Friendly visitor program

87. What is a good strategy for helping an elderly patient overcome feelings of low self-esteem related to chronic illness and loss of autonomy?

a. Praise the patient for any activities.
b. Tell the patient she has no reason to feel so depressed.
c. Provide opportunities for the patient to make decisions.
d. Encourage the patient to focus on positive factors.

88. Which of the following requests by a family member indicates a misunderstanding of Medicare/Medicaid rules regarding hospice care?

a. "Mother needs help bathing and washing her hair."
b. "Mother needs a speech therapist or occupational therapist to help her deal with her dysphagia."
c. "Mother needs a hospital bed with a trapeze."
d. "Mother needs to stay in the hospital when she becomes bedridden."

89. When determining the burden of proof for acts of negligence, how would risk management classify willfully providing inadequate care while disregarding the safety and security of another?

a. Negligent conduct
b. Gross negligence
c. Contributory negligence
d. Comparative negligence

90. A legal document that specifically designates someone to make decisions regarding medical and end-of-life care if a patient is mentally incompetent is a(n):

a. Advance directive
b. Do not resuscitate (DNR) order
c. Durable power of attorney
d. General power of attorney

91. An 80-year-old male has had post-herpetic neuralgia for 11 months, but his pain is increasingly intractable despite treatment with 10 hydrocodone tablets daily. He has coronary stents in place and takes warfarin. The patient is weak, somnolent, and lethargic, and eats and sleeps poorly. Modifying his pain management should include:

a. Weaning the patient from hydrocodone and starting gabapentin in slowly increasing doses
b. Discontinuing hydrocodone and starting a morphine pump
c. Weaning the patient from hydrocodone and starting biofeedback
d. Lowering the dose of hydrocodone and supplementing it with nonsteroidal anti-inflammatory drugs (NSAIDs)

92. A 78-year-old male with stage IV prostate cancer and moderate Alzheimer's disease is usually docile, but becomes very agitated and disruptive during mealtimes in the communal dining room of his residential care facility. The initial step to handling this problem is to:

a. Provide meals in the patient's room.
b. Encourage more participation by giving the patient meal choices.
c. Request a physician order for antipsychotic medication.
d. Observe the patient carefully to determine what triggers the agitation.

93. Fatigue that has no identifiable physiological purpose, and is unrelated to activity or exertion, is classified as:

a. Acute fatigue
b. Chronic fatigue
c. Secondary fatigue
d. Peripheral fatigue

94. A 56-year-old woman with advanced cervical cancer has bony metastasis and severe intractable bone pain. The most effective treatment is:

a. Radiation
b. Increased narcotic analgesia
c. Biofeedback
d. Adjuvant therapy with NSAIDs and tricyclic antidepressants

95. There is only one hospice bed available, but two patients need care, so the nurse recommends that one patient be transferred to another facility. The decision regarding which patient to transfer should be based on which ethical principle?

a. Nonmaleficence
b. Beneficence
c. Justice
d. Autonomy

96. A 42-year-old woman is receiving end-of-life care for stage IV breast cancer. She has developed a pronounced bronchial death rattle, which is distressing to her adolescent daughter and son. Death is expected within a few hours. Which of the following treatments is most indicated?

a. Glycopyrrolate or atropine subcutaneously
b. Morphine sulfate subcutaneously
c. Hyoscine hydrobromide (Scopolamine) transdermal patch
d. Oropharyngeal suctioning

97. The most common treatment for depression in those at the end of life is:

a. Psychotherapy
b. SSRIs
c. Tricyclic antidepressants
d. Stimulants, such as dextroamphetamine

98. When helping a dying patient complete a life review, the best approach is:

a. Ask yes/no questions so the patient doesn't tire.
b. Ask open-ended questions to elicit more information.
c. Direct questions to a close family member rather than the patient.
d. Use a standardized questionnaire.

99. An infant has died during an inter-hospital transfer, and the sobbing mother takes the infant in her arms and refuses to relinquish the child. Which is the most appropriate initial action?

a. Provide the mother a place to hold her child as long as she wants.
b. Ask family members to intervene.
c. Request that the hospital chaplain speak with the mother.
d. Explain to the mother the hospital procedures regarding death.

100. A patient's pain has been well controlled with morphine sulfate, extended release, but she has developed severe side effects and is being switched to an equianalgesic drug. The dosage of the new drug should be:

a. The equianalgesic dose
b. 25% above equianalgesic dose
c. 10% below equianalgesic dose
d. 25-50% below equianalgesic dose

101. Bereavement is:

a. A normal response to loss
b. The public expression of grief
c. The time period of mourning
d. A change of mood and feeling of sadness

102. A patient with chronic obstructive pulmonary disease (COPD) is dying. The patient is only comfortable lying supine with the head of the bed elevated to 60 degrees, but is experiencing sacral skin breakdown from friction and shear. The best solution is to:

a. Change the patient's position every two hours.
b. Apply a pressure-reducing mattress or mattress overlay.
c. Lower the patient's head to 30-45 degrees for half the time.
d. Apply a skin barrier to the sacral area.

103. After a patient talks to the doctor, the nurse enters the room and finds the patient shaking and distraught. Which is the nurse's best response?

a. "What's wrong?"
b. "Do you want me to call your family?"
c. "You are shaking and seem worried."
d. "You don't need to worry. Everything will be all right."

104. A 50-year-old man dying with cardiovascular disease is Catholic and asks to take final communion even though it is 2 a.m. The nurse should:

a. Tell the patient that no priest is available.
b. Ask the patient if he would be willing to see the Protestant chaplain who is on call.
c. Tell the patient the priest will be called at 7 a.m.
d. Contact the patient's priest or a priest on call for the institution and ask him to come right away.

105. A patient with ovarian cancer is receiving a starting dose of parenteral morphine 5 mg every 4 hours around the clock to control pain, but has required 5 rescue doses of supplementary opioids during the past 24 hours. The best action is to:

a. Increase the baseline opioid dose.
b. Change to a different opioid.
c. Institute opioid rotation.
d. Add adjuvant medications.

106. A 62-year-old homeless man hospitalized for AIDS is to be discharged, but has no place to go and no income. Which of the following is of primary importance in preparing for discharge?

a. Specific directions for medication or treatments, including side effects
b. Information sheets outlining signs for all risk factors
c. List of safe shelters and help in applying for welfare assistance or Social Security
d. Follow-up appointment dates, with physicians, labs, or other healthcare providers

107. What is the minimal urinary output per hour expected for an adult patient?

a. 20 mL
b. 30 mL
c. 40 mL
d. 50 mL

108. A Hispanic patient is admitted to the palliative care unit, and the nurse is doing the admission history, but the patient speaks very little English. What should the nurse do?

a. Ask the patient's 12-year-old son, who is fluent in English, to translate.
b. Use sign language and pictures to supplement questions.
c. Arrange for an interpreter.
d. Ask the patient's wife, who speaks fair English, to answer the questions for her husband.

109. An 80-year-old patient is dying of cancer and has been in and out of consciousness. The family should be encouraged to:

a. Go home, as the patient does not know they are present.
b. Talk to the patient, as hearing is usually the last sense to fail.
c. Offer the patient frequent sips of water to avoid dehydration.
d. Raise the head of the patient's bed if respirations become strained, to help the patient clear secretions.

110. The Confusion Assessment Method is a tool that covers nine factors related to mental status. This tool is used to assess:

a. Delirium
b. Alzheimer's disease
c. Substance abuse
d. Brain injury

111. The caregiver for a 60-year-old woman with amyotrophic lateral sclerosis (ALS) states that the patient frequently chokes on food. Which of the following foods is least likely to cause choking for this patient?

a. A cup of coffee
b. Moderately thick split pea soup
c. Soft white bread
d. Finger foods, such as hot dogs

112. A 40-year-old patient who suffered a traumatic brain injury is in a vegetative state and being maintained on life support. Prior to the accident, the patient was estranged from her husband, who has a healthcare power of attorney for the patient and is living separately. A decision regarding continuation of life support must be made, but the family members cannot agree. Who has the legal right to make the decision?

a. The patient's mother
b. The patient's 18-year-old daughter
c. The patient's estranged husband
d. The facility's ethics committee

113. A 48-year-old female patient has terminal ovarian cancer. She says that her doctor has misdiagnosed her and she wants to see a different doctor. Which stage of Elisabeth Kübler-Ross's stages of grief (death and dying) is she likely experiencing?

a. Anger
b. Denial
c. Depression
d. Bargaining

114. When assessing a patient's level of consciousness, the nurse reports that the patient appears sleepy and is inattentive. This is characterized as:

a. Clouded consciousness
b. Confusion
c. Lethargy
d. Stupor

115. A patient with amyotrophic lateral sclerosis (ALS) has been diagnosed with severe dehydration (>15% fluid loss). Typical symptoms include:

a. Dry mouth and increased thirst
b. Dizziness, lethargy, reduced skin turgor, and orthostatic hypotension
c. Resting hypotension, confusion, tachycardia, and oliguria
d. Marked hypotension and anuria, in addition to the symptoms above

116. In a problem-focused plan of care for a patient whose death is expected within 2-4 weeks, which of the following would take priority?

a. Provision of adequate nutrition and hydration
b. Pain control
c. Prevention of pressure injuries
d. Maintenance of mobility

117. A patient with end-stage renal disease exhibits the following: ventricular arrhythmia with increasing electrocardiography (ECG) changes; weakness with ascending paralysis and hyperreflexia; diarrhea; and increasing confusion. The patient most likely has:

a. Hyperkalemia
b. Hypokalemia
c. Hypocalcemia
d. Hypercalcemia

118. A 70-year-old male with chronic cirrhosis and hepatic failure has developed portal hypertension. Which is the most common complication of portal hypertension?

a. Jaundice
b. Blockage of the bile duct
c. Hemorrhage of esophageal varices
d. Abdominal distension

119. Beck's triad (increased central venous pressure with distended neck veins, muffled heart sounds, and hypotension) is indicative of which condition?

a. Myocardial infarction
b. Aortic valve prolapse
c. Cardiac tamponade
d. Pulmonary embolism

120. A 66-year-old male with Parkinson's disease, who is on Medicare, is being discharged with an open draining leg ulcer that he cannot care for independently because of poor vision. Prior to this hospitalization for an infected leg ulcer, he had lived alone with his 14-year-old grandson, who was placed in foster care while the patient was in the hospital. The best solution is:

a. Transferring the patient to an extended care facility
b. Keeping the patient in the hospital until the wound has healed
c. Teaching the man's 14-year-old grandson to do wound care
d. Making a referral to a home health agency to provide in-home care

121. If a peripheral neurolytic blockade results in inadequate denervation, a common side effect is:

a. Paralysis
b. Neuropathic pain
c. Nausea and vomiting
d. Horner's syndrome

122. A 78-year-old woman, who is dying of colon cancer, has had her pain well controlled with MS Contin, but she has become increasingly confused and lethargic as her condition deteriorates. The family asks if her pain medication should be altered. The best initial action is to:

a. Increase the dosage of pain medication.
b. Decrease the dosage of pain medication.
c. Discontinue pain medications.
d. Change to a different pain medication.

123. Cordotomy is recommended for which type of pain?

a. Intractable unilateral pain below T-5
b. Intractable bilateral pain below T-5
c. Intractable unilateral pain below C-5
d. Intractable bilateral pain below C-5

124. All of the following are necessary elements in a pain diary EXCEPT:

a. Medication name and dosage
b. Pain intensity prior to taking medication
c. Pain intensity after taking medication
d. Patient's mood prior to taking medication

125. When facilitating music therapy to help a patient relax, the most important criterion in the choice of music is:

a. Genre of music
b. Patient preference
c. Delivery system
d. Rhythm and beat

126. Stage 3 lymphedema is usually characterized by:

a. Unilateral pitting edema
b. Bilateral pitting edema
c. Unilateral hard, non-pitting edema
d. Bilateral hard, non-pitting edema

127. Post-mastectomy pain syndrome (PMPS) is characterized by:

a. Feeling of constriction, as well as burning, prickling, or numbness
b. Generalized musculoskeletal pain, stiffness, and fatigue
c. Paresthesia and severe unrelenting muscle pain
d. Unexplained diffuse burning pain

128. A patient with a large abdominal mass complains of deep, "squeezing" abdominal pain, and has nausea, vomiting, and periods of diaphoresis when the pain is intense. This type of pain is classified as:

a. Somatic
b. Referred
c. Neuropathic
d. Visceral

129. A patient is having trouble paying attention unless actively engaged, and her field of perception is narrow, as she is not observant of others or the activities around her. What degree of anxiety does this represent?

a. Mild
b. Moderate
c. Severe
d. Panic

130. With which of the following conditions does the patient tend to have fluctuating periods of confusion and disorientation, with disorganized thought processes, which usually worsen during the night?

a. Anxiety
b. Depression
c. Dementia
d. Delirium

131. All of the following emergent conditions often mimic signs of anxiety EXCEPT:

a. Hyperglycemia
b. Pulmonary embolus
c. Electrolyte imbalance
d. Hypoxia

132. A hospice patient has severe pain from pancreatic cancer, which has been well controlled with morphine, but is refusing the medication because it makes him drowsy and lethargic. The best initial action is to:

a. Have the patient continue to take the medication.
b. Provide a lower dose of the medication.
c. Change to an equianalgesic.
d. Use complementary therapies.

133. When a patient is provided with a structured education plan for pain management, detailed information should be presented to the patient:

a. Immediately after onset of any pain
b. After the pain is controlled
c. Upon the patient's request
d. Before pain management begins

134. Distraction as a pain management tool is most effective for:

a. Severe, acute pain
b. Chronic pain
c. Short periods of acute discomfort
d. Neuropathic pain

135. Which of the following should be restricted in the diet of a patient with hepatic cancer and ascites?

a. Calcium
b. Carbohydrates
c. Sodium
d. Protein

136. A palliative care patient has completed chemotherapy for breast cancer and develops a platelet count of 19, 500 mm^3. Common findings at this level of thrombocytopenia include all of the following EXCEPT:

a. Nasal bleeding
b. Excessive menstrual flow
c. Petechiae
d. Gastrointestinal hemorrhage

137. A hospice patient nearing death should be offered food and fluids until:

a. The patient loses consciousness.
b. The patient stops showing interest.
c. The patient begins artificial feeding and hydration.
d. The patient becomes lethargic, sleeping much of the time.

138. A patient has entered palliative care after treatment for leukemia that included chemotherapy. The patient's white blood count is 5,300, and the absolute neutrophil count is 526 mm^3. The patient is at risk for:

a. Infection
b. Thromboembolism
c. Spontaneous fracture
d. Bleeding

139. Opioid-induced nausea and vomiting is best treated with:

a. Scopolamine
b. Metoclopramide
c. Phenothiazines
d. Haloperidol

140. The sites most commonly invaded by metastatic cancers are the:

a. Lungs, liver, and bones
b. Brain and bones
c. Adrenal glands and bones
d. Peritoneum and bones

141. All of the following are nonpharmacologic methods of relieving dyspnea EXCEPT:

a. Position of comfort
b. Rapid completion of tasks to maximize resting time
c. Cooling fan directed at face
d. Breathing exercises (pursed-lip and diaphragmatic breathing)

142. Patients with constant severe pain should receive pain medication:

a. When pain breaks through
b. On demand
c. Routinely around the clock
d. Four times daily

143. The antidiarrheal medication most indicated for secretory diarrhea associated with HIV/AIDS is:

a. Octreotide
b. Loperamide
c. Codeine sulfate
d. Diphenoxylate

144. A patient with end-stage renal disease has developed uremia and severe generalized pruritus. The best preventive is:

a. Phosphate binders
b. Dialysis
c. Topical phenol solution
d. Antihistamines

145. Right-sided heart failure is characterized by which of the following?

a. Pulmonary edema
b. Hypoxemia
c. Paroxysmal nocturnal dyspnea
d. Jugular vein distention

146. A patient with brain metastasis has sudden onset of a generalized seizure. The most common initial treatment is:

a. Phenytoin
b. Phenobarbital
c. Diazepam
d. Corticosteroids

147. A patient with stage IV lung cancer develops progressive dyspnea; facial swelling; edema of the neck, arms, hands, and thorax; distended jugular, temporal, and arm veins; visual disturbances; headache; and altered mental status. The most likely diagnosis is:

a. Syndrome of inappropriate secretion of antidiuretic hormone (SIADH)
b. Pulmonary embolism (PE)
c. Superior vena cava syndrome (SVCS)
d. Spinal cord compression

148. For hospice patients, hypnosis is most effective for use with:

a. Somatic pain
b. Neuropathic pain
c. Visceral pain
d. Procedural pain

149. A palliative care patient with recurrent breast cancer has developed a right pleural effusion and is to have a thoracentesis to relieve dyspnea. Which of the following is the most effective patient position for the procedure?

a. Sitting, leaning forward
b. Prone
c. Side-lying on the right
d. Side-lying on the left

150. A patient with ovarian cancer suddenly develops severe nausea and vomiting in large volumes. Her abdomen is painful and rigid, bowel sounds are diminished, and she feels short of breath. She has no fever. She reports that she has had only very small bowel movements recently. The most likely diagnosis is:

a. Fecal impaction
b. Obstruction of the small intestine
c. Obstruction of the colon
d. Peritonitis

Answers and Explanations

1. A: Support surface material should provide at least an inch of support, when in use, under areas to be protected; if there is less than an inch of support, the material has bottomed out. Check the support material by sliding a hand underneath the overlay in the area where the patient has a pressure injury to determine how much support there is. Static support surfaces are appropriate for patients who can change position without increasing pressure to a wound. Dynamic support surfaces are best for those who need assistance to move, or when static pressure devices provide less than an inch of support.

2. C: Midazolam is a very rapid, short-acting benzodiazepine used for terminal sedation. It can be administered intravenously or subcutaneously. Pentobarbital is a long-acting barbiturate that is administered intravenously or subcutaneously, while propofol is an anesthetic agent with very rapid onset that requires continuous intravenous (IV) infusion. Lorazepam is a short-acting benzodiazepine that can be administered orally, buccally, intravenously, or subcutaneously. Terminal sedation is indicated when the patient has severe symptoms that cannot be relieved, such as intractable pain, severe nausea and vomiting, feeling of suffocation, or seizures.

3. B: In the last stages of amyotrophic lateral sclerosis (ALS), profound muscle weakness leads to an inability to breathe independently, and patients require mechanical ventilation to breathe. Some patients sign an advance directive indicating that they do not wish to be placed on a ventilator. Some ALS patients may exhibit signs of dementia in the later stages of the disease. Weight loss is common as patients have increasing difficulty chewing and swallowing. Slurred speech tends to occur early in the disease process.

4. A: Acetaminophen (325-650 mg every 4-6 hours) or ibuprofen (200-800 mg every 4 hours) is commonly used to treat temperatures above 38.3 °C (101 °F). Aspirin is not recommended for control of fever because of possible adverse effects. Alcohol baths are no longer recommended and should be avoided. A cold bath may trigger shivering and increase patient discomfort. A bath in tepid water may help reduce a high temperature that does not respond to medications. In some cases, elevated temperature may indicate dehydration, so providing fluids is also important.

5. D: Because myelosuppression (a decrease in bone marrow activity) can result in anemia, and thereby increase the risk of inadequate oxygen supply to tissues, a high-protein diet is advised. Other effects of myelosuppression include neutropenia (a decrease in the white blood cells known as neutrophils), which increases the risk of infection, and thrombocytopenia (a decrease in the number of platelets in the blood), which increases the risk of bleeding. Patients should avoid activities that might stress the body or result in complications. Therefore, strenuous activities, shaving, and alcohol consumption should be avoided. The degree of myelosuppression varies depending on the type of chemotherapeutic agent used. For example, irinotecan (used to treat colon and rectal cancer) results in neutropenia, while fluorouracil results in suppression of red blood cells, white blood cells, and platelets.

6. A: Pain in the flank areas and lack of bladder distention suggest that the cause of the urinary retention is an upper urinary tract obstruction resulting from spread of the ovarian cancer. If the ureters are obstructed and urine is unable to drain, the patient will develop uremia, which is associated with hyperkalemia. With bladder infection or opioid-induced deficiency of detrusor muscle contractions, the bladder should fill normally and become distended, with pain usually felt in the suprapubic area.

7. B: While in some cases infections may be allowed to run their course in hospice patients nearing death, this MRSA infection is increasing the patient's pain, so antibiotics should be used to provide palliation, and the pain management should be modified so the patient is more comfortable. Additionally, MRSA poses a threat to caregivers because it is easily transmitted by contact, so reducing the risk to others can be factored into the decision to treat the infection. Caregivers should be advised to use both standard and contact precautions.

8. C: The nurse should remain supportive and nonjudgmental. The response "I'll stay with him, and you can come and go as you feel comfortable" supports the daughter's stated desire while leaving open the opportunity for her to spend time with her father during the death vigil. People react in different ways to death. Many people have never witnessed the process of dying, or have never seen a deceased person, and therefore may be frightened by the prospect. While many people find comfort in being with a dying friend or family member, this decision should never be imposed on anyone.

9. D: Pain appears to be driving this patient to suicidal ideation, so the best response is to first directly address the comment to determine the severity of suicidal ideation by asking if the patient has a plan to hurt himself. After the immediate risk assessment, the nurse should find ways to alleviate the cause of this patient's distress by offering to work together to find better ways to manage the pain. Many people fear pain more than death, and patients have a right (legal and moral) to be free of pain at the end of life. The nurse should assess the type, frequency, and duration of pain and current pain management. In some cases, a change to a stronger medication, such as an opioid, or the addition of adjuvant medications, may be indicated. Suicidal ideation should be reported to the attending physician, and the caregivers should be alerted.

10. D: Tremors and jerking movements are consistent with opioid-induced myoclonus. Myoclonus may be caused by a range of drugs, including opioids and quinolones. The patient is being treated with fentanyl, which is a synthetic opioid. In this case, changing to an equianalgesic should relieve symptoms in 1-2 days. If the myoclonus is mild, a benzodiazepine at bedtime may prevent the muscle twitching from awakening the patient. While similar symptoms may occur with brain metastasis, it is unlikely that this metastasis would occur with prostate cancer. Anxiety may also produce similar symptoms, but these would be less pronounced and less likely to cause jerking during sleep. Damage to the spine would produce different symptoms.

11. B: The patient's activity immediately prior to the episode of syncope can help to determine the cause. For example, if the patient was leaning down to pick up something and stood up abruptly, this could trigger syncope. Once the circumstances are established, the nurse should question the patient in more detail because many factors could be involved, including sleep deprivation, malnutrition, medications, alcohol use, and severe anxiety. It is important to get information about the duration of the episode because syncopal episodes are usually short with fairly rapid recovery after the episode.

12. C: Clinical signs such as pallor, orthostatic hypotension, and tachycardia provide the most effective initial evaluation of the extent of a hemorrhage. Readings of hemoglobin and hematocrit may remain stable following a hemorrhage because red blood cells and plasma are lost in proportional amounts, though this would change over time. Arterial PO_2 also may remain stable initially, so it would not be a good indicator of the seriousness of the hemorrhage.

13. A: These findings are consistent with disseminated intravascular coagulation (DIC), which is a secondary disorder that is triggered by another disorder, such as trauma, congenital heart disease, necrotizing enterocolitis, sepsis, or severe viral infections. The patient is suffering from infection and sepsis, which put her at risk for DIC. DIC causes both coagulation and hemorrhage through a complex series of events, including trauma that causes tissue factor (transmembrane glycoprotein) to enter the circulation and bind with coagulation factors, thereby triggering the coagulation cascade. This stimulates thrombin to convert fibrinogen to fibrin, causing aggregation and destruction of platelets and forming clots that can be disseminated throughout the intravascular system. Red blood cells are also destroyed.

14. B: Sudden acute unilateral pleuritic pain, dyspnea, tachypnea, tachycardia, and slight cough, along with unilateral decreased breath sounds, are consistent with pneumothorax, which can occur with lung cancer as the tumor erodes through the surface of the lung. If air continues to escape, a tension pneumothorax may occur with tracheal deviation and marked hemodynamic compromise. A small pneumothorax may heal spontaneously over 1-2 weeks, although a chest tube may be inserted for a larger pneumothorax. Tension pneumothorax requires immediate needle decompression and insertion of chest tube.

15. B: Pursed-lip breathing is one of the breathing exercises recommended for patients with chronic obstructive pulmonary disease (COPD). This kind of breathing, which involves breathing in through the nose and a longer exhalation through pursed lips, helps prevent the small airways in the lungs from collapsing so that trapped air can be exhaled. It also slows the patient's breathing rate and helps the patient to relax. Inspiratory muscle training requires inhaling against resistance through a special device to improve muscle strength; this training can improve the COPD patient's endurance when exercising or doing other physical activity. Paced walking involves matching inhalation and exhalation to paces; for example, a patient may breathe in for two paces and out for four. Diaphragmatic breathing helps to improve alveolar ventilation and may help to expel air as well, since the diaphragm muscles are strengthened and used more effectively.

16. D: The heart sound rhythm that is categorized as S3, heard with the patient lying on the left side, may indicate heart failure or left ventricular failure in older adults. An opening snap is an unusual high-pitched sound that is caused by mitral valve stenosis from rheumatic heart disease. An ejection click is a brief high-pitched sound occurring immediately after S1, and may indicate a septal defect. Friction rub is a dry, grating sound heard in systole and diastole with pericarditis.

17. A: Chronic renal failure is characterized by hyperkalemia rather than hypokalemia**.** Chronic renal failure occurs when the kidneys are unable to filter and excrete wastes, concentrate urine, and maintain electrolyte balance because of hypoxic conditions, kidney disease, or obstruction of the urinary tract. It results first in azotemia (increase in nitrogenous waste in the blood) and then in uremia (nitrogenous wastes cause toxic symptoms). Metabolic acidosis and sodium and fluid retention occur, as well as anemia. When more than 50% of the functional renal capacity is destroyed, the kidneys can no longer carry out necessary functions, and progressive deterioration begins over months or years.

18. A: Left-hemisphere strokes often result in right-sided paresis or paralysis and aphasia, which may be expressive, receptive, or global. Patients may also experience short-term memory loss and difficulty learning new materials. Brainstem strokes may impair respiratory and cardiac function. Cerebellar strokes may cause ataxia, nausea and vomiting, headaches, and dizziness or vertigo. Right-hemisphere strokes result in left paresis or paralysis and left-sided neglect (lack of perception of things on the left side), as well as short-term memory loss and depression.

19. D: Variant angina, also known as Prinzmetal angina, results from spasms of the coronary arteries. This form of angina is not caused by physical or emotional stress, but can be associated with intake of nicotine, alcohol, or some other stimulant such as cocaine. Variant angina frequently occurs cyclically at the same time each day, usually while the person is at rest. Stable angina episodes usually last for less than 5 minutes and are fairly predictable, exercise-induced episodes caused by atherosclerotic lesions blocking more than 75% of the lumen of the affected coronary artery. Unstable angina is a progression of coronary artery disease and occurs with a change in the pattern of stable angina. Esophageal varices usually cause no symptoms before bleeding.

20. B: Femur fractures may result from preexisting osteoporosis or from a traumatic injury, such as a fall. Additionally, some types of cancer, such as breast cancer and prostate cancer, may metastasize to the femur, weakening it and resulting in fracture. Treatment varies but may include analgesia and surgical repair, as well as radiation to shrink the underlying tumor with metastasis. The extent of treatment depends on the patient's condition and life expectancy, in conjunction with the patient's wishes.

21. C: Haloperidol is a common cause of extrapyramidal symptoms. These effects are the result of drug influence on the parts of the nervous system that control involuntary movement and help coordinate voluntary movements. Extrapyramidal symptoms include:

- Akinesia (inability to start movement)
- Akathisia (inability to stop movement)
- Dystonia (extreme and uncontrolled muscle contraction, torticollis, flexing, and twisting)

The most common extrapyramidal condition caused by antipsychotic agents is tardive dyskinesia. Individuals with this condition are unable to control their movements, and display tics, lip smacking, and eye blinking. The term *tardive* refers to the delayed onset of the symptoms. Even after the discontinuation of a drug, extrapyramidal side effects may still be present.

22. A: When treating anxiety in a geriatric patient, short-acting benzodiazepines, such as lorazepam or temazepam, are usually well tolerated, while tricyclic antidepressants and β-adrenergic agents may cause adverse effects. Short-acting benzodiazepines are also the drugs of choice for pediatric patients. Long-acting benzodiazepines may result in confusion in the elderly. If benzodiazepines are not effective, patients may respond to selective serotonin reuptake inhibitors (SSRIs) or low-dose antihistamines. Low-dose antihistamines have a sedating effect and can be especially useful for treating anxiety in geriatric patients who also have respiratory dysfunction.

23. B: Peripherally inserted central catheters (PICCs) are frequently used for intravenous (IV) infusions that will continue for several weeks or months (intermediate-term). PICC lines are used for chemotherapy and are inserted in one of the arms, usually above the elbow. Non-tunneled central catheters are used for short-term therapy of less than 6 weeks. Tunneled central catheters are inserted when patients require long-term intravenous therapy, as these devices can remain in place for many years. Implantable ports are also used primarily for long-term IV therapy. Once implanted, the ports require little care and are easily accessed.

24. A: Patients with opioid tolerance do not exhibit an increase in side effects. On the contrary, one of the characteristics of opioid tolerance is that patients experience a very low incidence of side effects or have very mild side effects. Other characteristics include complaints of pain that is much more severe than usually associated with the patient's condition or disease. Additionally, the patient tends to need excessively high doses of the medication to control pain and may request pain medications much more frequently as pain breaks through. If patients require larger and larger doses to relieve pain, then changing to a different medication is usually indicated.

25. D: Acupuncture is probably the most effective adjunct therapy for pain and is widely used. Music therapy may reduce the need for analgesia by helping the patient relax. Therapeutic touch has also been widely used, and many patients feel it relieves pain, even though recent studies suggest that it is not effective. Therapeutic touch is passive, requiring little involvement of the patient, and patients may find it comforting. Massage can relieve muscle discomfort and promote relaxation.

26. B: Nonsteroidal anti-inflammatory drugs (NSAIDs) are contraindicated as co-adjuvants with corticosteroids because they have similar side effects and can increase the risk of gastrointestinal irritation and bleeding. NSAIDs may be used as sole analgesia initially to treat mild to moderate pain and are used as adjuvant drugs with opioids at steps 2 or 3 of the analgesic ladder. NSAIDs provide an anti-inflammatory effect and are especially effective for reducing bone pain. While NSAIDS do not produce dependence or addiction and may reduce the need for opioids, they are associated with many adverse effects.

27. A: Withholding food and fluids in the dying patient can lead to increased ketones, which elevate levels of endorphins and lead to an electrolyte imbalance that results in analgesia and decreased pain and discomfort. Respiratory distress may lessen because of a decrease in pulmonary fluids. Nausea and vomiting can result if food and fluids are provided to a patient whose digestive system is slowing down. As the kidney function fails, fluids can cause increased peripheral edema and congestive heart failure, adding to a patient's discomfort and risk of developing pressure injuries.

28. C: Opioids pose a risk of urinary retention, especially in older males with an enlarged prostate. Urinary retention may also occur when patients are taking tricyclic antidepressants along with an opioid. Patients may develop increased smooth muscle tone, which can cause bladder spasms. However, in some cases, this increased tone affects the sphincter, leading to urinary retention. Myoclonus can occur with all opioids but is related to dose and toxicity. pruritus is most common with morphine. Delirium usually results from a combination of problems, such as electrolyte disorders or organ failure, along with opioids.

29. D: Bisphosphonates are commonly used as adjuvant drugs to relieve osteolytic bone pain since they can help slow the breakdown of bone. Tricyclic antidepressants are used to treat burning neuropathic pain and to relieve insomnia or depression, while anticonvulsants are used for sharp, shooting, shock-like neuropathic pain. Corticosteroids have broad use for bone pain, neuropathic pain, visceral pain, and cord compression, as well as pain crisis.

30. D: A psychological response to grief can include imitating a deceased spouse's behavior. Other psychological responses include anger, guilt, suspicion, and other emotional responses, as well as idealization of or ambivalence about the deceased. Physical responses might include insomnia, nervousness, palpitations, crying, and weight gain or loss. A spiritual response to grief may involve fear of God, anger at God, or focusing on beliefs about the afterlife. Sociocultural responses to grief include the death rituals or the attitudes about life-prolonging measures that are normative in a particular society, community, or group.

31. A: Patients normally stop taking fluids as they near death, resulting in dehydration and drying of the mucous membranes of the mouth. Frequent mouth care, including moistening of the mucous membranes, can alleviate mouth discomfort. Mouth care includes cleaning with a soft toothbrush or sponge swab, rinsing the mouth with water, misting with a spray bottle, or placing loose, damp gauze over the patient's mouth. The patient's lips should be lubricated to prevent cracking. The mouth may be swabbed with artificial saliva, such as Salivart.

32. B: Decreased cardiac output and intravascular volume result in tachycardia, not bradycardia, as the heart attempts to compensate. Patients become hypotensive and peripheral and/or central cyanosis occurs as the body attempts to conserve the blood supply for the internal organs. When the blood supply to the skin decreases, there is less oxygen, and the skin surface may appear bluish. The skin may also feel cool to the touch. As death nears, mottling (large patches that appear purple or reddish-blue) may appear, beginning with the soles of the feet, earlobes, and knees.

33. A: When evaluating a patient for pain management, the initial objective should be to identify treatable causes of the pain, such as improper positioning or infection. Addressing the cause of the pain may eliminate the need for pain management or may alter the course of pain management. Once treatable causes are identified and eliminated, if possible, then the level of pain and the patient's physical and psychological status can be evaluated in order to choose an effective pain medication or pain management program to meet the individual's needs.

34. C: Gynecomastia is a common adverse effect of androgen-deprivation therapy with diethylstilbestrol (DES) because the normal balance of estrogen and testosterone is impaired. DES is a synthetic estrogen that results in breast enlargement. Other androgen-deprivation methods include orchiectomy, or the administration of luteinizing hormone-releasing hormone (LHRH) or other drugs that inhibit androgen, such as aminoglutethimide. All of these treatments may result in decreased libido. Hot flashes may occur after orchiectomy. Bone pain may occur in prostate cancer patients who also have bony metastases; however, this would not result from DES treatment.

35. C: Metoclopramide is used to relieve hiccups associated with gastric distention since it acts to empty the stomach contents. Agents containing simethicone/dimethicone may also relieve distention and relieve hiccups. Baclofen or chlorpromazine is also used to treat intractable hiccups. Omeprazole would be appropriate to treat prolonged hiccupping caused by gastroesophageal reflux. Other medications, such as haloperidol, are sometimes given to relax the diaphragm muscle. Conservative approaches include eating a teaspoon of sugar or chewing on crushed ice. Hiccups may result from gastric distention, diaphragm irritation, pancreatitis, corticosteroids, renal failure, brain tumors, and infection.

36. A: Palliative care can begin when a patient is diagnosed with a life-threatening disease, such as advanced cancer or amyotrophic lateral sclerosis (ALS). In some cases, patients with serious chronic diseases, such as chronic obstructive pulmonary disease (COPD), may be referred for palliative care even though death does not appear imminent. A patient request for palliative care is not adequate unless that patient has an appropriate diagnosis. Palliative care may be supportive in the early stages but intensifies as a patient's condition deteriorates.

37. D: An opioid-naive patient is one who has not been taking daily opioids routinely, while an opioid-tolerant patient is one who has been taking daily opioids routinely (for at least a week) at doses equivalent to 60 mg morphine (PO) daily, generally to control chronic and severe pain. The status of a patient in relation to opioids is important when symptoms escalate or new symptoms develop because opioid tolerance may lead to decreased drug effectiveness, although some adverse effects, such as respiratory depression, may actually decrease.

38. B: When a patient is nearing death, the most important consideration is comfort, even if this means that some routine patient care, such as turning the patient, must be set aside. The patient should be allowed to lie undisturbed as much as possible. The process of transferring a patient to another bed may cause discomfort and distress.

39. A: Removing the Foley catheter and substituting disposable underwear is not a viable option given the presence of the coccygeal pressure injury. Because sediment builds up on a catheter over time and can irritate the bladder, routinely changing of the catheter may relieve symptoms. Inserting a catheter in a smaller size or with a smaller balloon can also result in less irritation to the bladder lining and reduce spasms. Oxybutynin can be effective in reducing spasms if more conservative methods are unsuccessful.

40. B: Under the American Nurses Association (ANA) Code of Ethics for Nurses, autonomy and self-determination are viewed within the broad context of diverse cultures. The idea of individualism is less important in some cultures, so the nurse must respect and appreciate the patient's right to be guided by her family. Trying to convince the patient to assert herself may just lead to emotional conflict. This is not an appropriate concern for the ethics committee, as the woman is not being forced to comply with family decisions, but chooses to do so.

41. A: According to Bowen family systems theory, this would be a classic example of a family triangle dynamic. Bowen family systems theory considers the relationship between three people to be a basic emotional unit that has great stability, since tensions between any two members in the triad are mediated by the presence of the third party. The resulting dynamic often involves two of the people in agreement, with the third person disagreeing, or feeling left out. Bowen family systems theory suggests that a person be understood in terms of the interdependent family unit, where a change in one person's behavior will affect the others in the family. Other concepts include:

- Projection within a family: Emotional problems may be passed from parent to child.
- Transmission (multigenerational): Small differences in conscious and unconscious transmission from parents to children allow for a differentiation between siblings.
- Emotional isolation: Reducing or eliminating family contact may be used as a way to deal with unresolved conflicts.

42. D: Collaboration requires an assertive rather than an unassertive approach, with ideas stated in a calm, nonthreatening manner. Other collaborative skills include:

- Casual conversation: Asking open-ended questions, asking about others' work, or commenting on someone's contributions helps to establish a relationship.
- Competence in public speaking: Collaboration requires that a nurse be comfortable speaking and presenting ideas to groups of people in a credible manner.
- Competence in writing: The written word remains a critical component of communication, and the nurse should be able to communicate clearly and grammatically.

43. C: Asking "What would you like to include in your plan of care?" gives the patient and family members a chance to be active participants in the development of the plan. They should be included from the beginning and encouraged to voice preferences and opinions. While patients and family members should be encouraged to ask questions, and should be notified of necessary changes to the plan, this type of input usually occurs after the plan has been developed and does not give them control in the process.

44. B: The economic aspects of care are not part of the Domains of Quality Palliative Care, which serve as a guide for the provision of care in palliative care programs. Palliative care can be provided in a variety of settings, including the home and hospital. The purpose of the guidelines is to promote quality care and facilitate partnerships and collaboration to meet patient needs. The domains are:

- Structure and processes of care
- Physical aspects of care
- Psychological and psychiatric aspects of care
- Social aspects of care
- Spiritual, religious, and existential aspects of care
- Cultural aspects of care
- Care of the patient nearing the end of life
- Ethical and legal aspects of care

45. D: A stool laxative or softener should be taken daily to prevent or treat constipation associated with opioid use. If patients cannot tolerate oral medications, then methylnaltrexone administered subcutaneously may relieve constipation. Bulking agents should be avoided because they can increase constipation and impaction if the patient is not able to drink adequate fluids, as is common with debilitated patients. Reducing the dose of the opioid may increase the patient's pain, so treating the adverse effect is more important than removing the cause. While adequate fluid intake is preferred, forcing fluids may increase a patient's discomfort and cause nausea.

46. A: Steps to conflict resolution include:

- Allow both sides to present their side of the conflict without bias, maintaining a focus on opinions rather than individuals.
- Encourage cooperation through negotiation and compromise.
- Maintain the focus, providing guidance to keep the discussions on track and avoid arguments.
- Evaluate the need for renegotiation, a formal resolution process, or third-party involvement.

The best time for conflict resolution is when differences emerge but before open conflict and hardening of positions. The nurse must pay close attention to the people involved, try to understand the problem, listen carefully, and reassure those involved that their points of view are understood and respected.

47. B: Sharps should never be disposed of in glass containers because the glass may break. While state laws vary slightly, in general, clear containers (plastic or glass) should always be avoided. Opaque puncture-resistant hard plastic or metal containers are acceptable, but should be clearly labeled with "Biohazard," "Do not recycle," or "Sharps," according to state guidelines. The lids should be secured with tape prior to disposal, which should be done in accordance with regulations. Most states allow disposal of such containers in household trash.

48. B: During the death vigil, the nurse should stay with the family and sit quietly, allowing them to talk, cry, or interact if they desire. Other guidelines include:

- Avoid platitudes such as "His suffering will be over soon."
- Avoid judgmental reactions to what family members say or do, and realize that anger, fear, guilt, and irrational behavior are normal responses to acute grief and stress.
- Show caring by touching the patient and encouraging the family to do the same. Note: Touching the hands, arms, or shoulders of family members can provide comfort, but follow cues from the family and avoid hugging, which may be misconstrued.
- Provide referrals to support groups if available.

49. D: The patient's inability to understand oral instructions and lack of interest in illustrations suggest that he may be a kinesthetic learner, so the nurse should allow the patient to handle the equipment and practice. Kinesthetic learners understand information best by handling, doing, and practicing with minimal directions and hands-on experience. Other learning styles include visual and auditory learning. Visual learners take in and understand new information by seeing and reading. Teaching strategies for visual learners include:

- Provide written directions and picture guides, or demonstrate procedures.
- Use charts and diagrams.
- Provide photos and videos.

Auditory learners learn best by listening and talking. Teaching strategies for auditory learners include:

- Explain procedures while demonstrating, and have the learner repeat.
- Plan extra time to discuss and answer questions.
- Provide audiotapes.

50. B: Islamic tradition forbids cremation of the body. Traditionally, the body is bathed with water (with the genitals covered), usually by a spouse, parent of a minor child, or members of the family who are of the same gender. The washed body is wrapped in a shroud, usually made from plain white cloth, with three pieces used for males and five for females. Funeral prayers (*Janazah*) are said during a gathering of people to honor the dead. Burial should take place within 24 hours of the death.

51. A: Cheyne-Stokes respirations are characterized by hypernea (deep breaths) alternating with apnea (cessation of breath). As the lungs become less effective and more congested, gas exchange is poor, and carbon dioxide levels increase. This increase usually triggers respiration, but as brain function decreases, this function is impaired, so respirations may deepen and then become more shallow and irregular, with periods of apnea that may last for up to a minute in a repeating cycle. Kussmaul respirations are characterized by labored, gasping breaths, and are associated with metabolic acidosis. Tachypnea refers to a respiratory pattern of rapid, shallow breaths, while bradypnea refers to a pattern of breathing much slower than normal.

52. C: The symptoms described are typical of oral candidiasis (thrush), which is common with cancer patients. Nystatin oral suspension is often used to treat the condition and relieve symptoms. If candidiasis persists or does not respond well to oral suspension or troches, then a systemic medication such as fluconazole may be indicated. Providing good mouth care and keeping the mucous membranes moist can help to prevent candidiasis. Dentures should be removed during the night and after meals for cleansing. In some patients, the white lesions may be absent, but the tongue may be reddened and irritated.

53. D: Acetaminophen is contraindicated in patients with liver disease, as toxicity may occur, especially if the patient is alcoholic. Acetaminophen is commonly used as an adjuvant for mild to moderate pain but can also be used with more severe pain, especially if the patient cannot tolerate nonsteroidal anti-inflammatory drugs (NSAIDs). Acetaminophen rarely causes gastrointestinal irritation and does not affect platelets, so it does not increase the danger of bleeding. Acetaminophen can be used in patients who have a hypersensitivity to aspirin.

54. A: This statement indicates that the caregiver is blaming the patient for problems common to a dying patient rather than focusing on the problem of incontinence, and this can indicate the possibility of abuse in which the caregiver essentially "punishes" the patient. Caregivers, especially those involved in long-term care, often express that they wish the patient would die. They may feel that the patient is suffering, or they are exhausted from caregiving. Feeling tired and overwhelmed is a common problem associated with caregiving but should not be read as a warning of potential abuse.

55. C: Helping the family make funeral arrangements is outside the expected formal closure activities and responsibilities of the hospice nurse. However, making a final visit to the family after a patient's death can help the family find closure. Other appropriate activities include telephoning family members and sending cards or messages of condolence. In some cases, family members may want to establish long-term relationships with healthcare providers, but this can establish a dependent relationship that may prove detrimental and should be avoided.

56. B: Tracer methodology looks at the continuum of care a patient receives from admission to post-discharge. A patient is selected to be "traced," and the medical record serves as a guide. Tracer methodology uses the experience of the selected patient to evaluate the processes in place through documents and interviews. Root-cause analysis (RCA) is a retrospective attempt to determine the cause of an event, often a sentinel event such as an unexpected death, or a cluster of events. Root-cause analysis involves interviews, observations, and review of medical records. Family and staff surveys may provide helpful but less detailed information.

57. A: For patients already receiving morphine, increasing the dose by 2.5 mg may relieve the sensation of breathlessness. Opioid-naive patients may benefit from a dose of 5 mg morphine orally every 4 hours. Providing oxygen usually only provides some relief if the dyspnea is associated with hypoxia, such as with patients with chronic obstructive pulmonary disease (COPD), and patients may feel that the oxygen is helpful, thereby reducing their anxiety. Elevating the head of the bed should be done routinely for patients with dyspnea, but that alone may be ineffective for severe dyspnea.

58. D: According to the Dying Person's Bill of Rights, every patient has a right to hope for the best outcome and to participate in religious or spiritual activities of their choice, so the correct response would be to ask, "What can I do to help?" The nurse should not express an opinion that the healing is unrealistic, nor put the burden on the patient by saying, "If you believe." Patients have a right to seek spiritual guidance and healing without a doctor's permission. Traditional Hmong families may shun Western medicine and rely solely on healers, while Christian Hmong may rely only on Western medicine. However, many Hmong people straddle both the traditional and Western worlds.

59. C: Generally, hospice programs require patients to have a "do not resuscitate" (DNR) order and a diagnosis of a life-threatening disease. These criteria alone are not sufficient, however, since patients with longer life expectancies can be referred to palliative care programs. Severe intractable pain may be one problem hospice addresses, but pain can occur in patients who do not have a life-threatening disease.

60. D: While Foley catheters pose a risk of increased infection, this is not a primary concern in the dying patient, and insertion of the Foley catheter to control incontinence can provide a measure of comfort and may reduce skin irritation. While disposable underwear and skin barriers may be the first choice when a patient is more able to move during the earlier stages, turning and moving the patient to apply and remove underwear and skin barriers may increase discomfort in the later stages of dying.

61. A: Whole medical systems are based on coherent medical theories and practices that were developed before—or as an alternative to—standard Western medical theory and practice. According to the National Center for Complementary and Alternative Medicine (NCCAM), whole medical systems include traditional Chinese medicine (which uses acupuncture and herbal medications), Ayurvedic medicine, homeopathy, and naturopathy. Meditation is an example of a mind-body practice; other examples of this include tai chi, chi gong, yoga, and guided imagery. Biologically based natural product practices include the use of food, vitamins, or nutrition for healing. Manipulative/body-based programs include massage or spinal manipulation, such as chiropractic treatment. NAACM also recognizes other complementary and alternative medical practices, such as energy therapies (therapeutic touch, Reiki, chi gong, and bioelectromagnetic-based practices) and movement therapies (Pilates, Rolfing, the Feldenkrais method, the Alexander technique, and Trager).

62. A: The best readability level is grade 6. The average American reads most effectively at the sixth- to eighth-grade level (regardless of education achieved), and research shows that even people with much higher reading skills learn medical and health information most effectively when the material is presented at this readability level. A third-grade level would be too simplified for most native speakers but might be appropriate for immigrant populations with limited English.

63. B: The nurse should not disclose personal information, such as an impending divorce, because this establishes a social relationship that interferes with the professional role of the nurse. Small tokens of appreciation that can be shared with other staff, such as a box of chocolates, are usually acceptable (depending upon the policy of the institution), but almost any other personal gifts (e.g., jewelry, money, or clothes) should be declined. Helping a patient place a phone call is not a boundary issue. Touching should be used with care since some kinds of physical contact, such as hugging, may be misconstrued as inappropriate touching.

64. D: Bed rest is not an appropriate treatment for dependent edema because activity may aid venous return and maintain muscle tone and strength. Treatment for dependent edema includes providing skin care, elevating the legs, applying graded elastic compression stockings, and administering a diuretic. Edema is rated on a 1-4 point scale:

- 1+ Slight pitting to about 2 mm (persists 10-15 seconds)
- 2+ Moderate pitting to about 4 mm (persists 10-15 seconds)
- 3+ Moderate or severe pitting to about 6 mm (persists >1 minute)
- 4+ Severe pitting to 8 mm or more (persists 2-5 minutes)

65. D: Self-determined life closure empowers patients to make decisions about end-of-life care. While advance directives and a "do not resuscitate" (DNR) request may contribute to self-determined life closure, the most important factor is ensuring that the patient's wishes are honored. In some cases, when a patient is no longer able to make decisions, others might make decisions that are at odds with the patient's wishes, either because they are unaware of those wishes or because they hold different opinions and beliefs about proper care. In self-determined life closure, caregivers and healthcare providers know the patients' wishes related to end-of life care, such as pain control, hospitalization, and cardiopulmonary resuscitation (CPR), through either advance directives or discussions, and ensure that the patients' preferences are respected.

66. A: A child life specialist has a broad knowledge of child development and has expertise in developmental assessments. This specialist works with families, prepares children for painful or unpleasant procedures, and facilitates therapeutic play. A child life specialist addresses the unique needs, both physical and emotional, of children of all ages. Additionally, child life specialists can serve as resources for other healthcare providers and families, helping them learn more about the needs and care of children. Child life specialists are trained in stress reduction techniques to reduce anxiety in children and their families.

67. C: Initially, the physician must certify that a patient who is eligible for Medicare A is terminal, with a life expectancy of 6 months or less (two 90-day periods), but if the patient remains alive, the physician can extend coverage by authorizing care every 60 days. The goal is to maintain the patient in the home environment with home health aides, homemakers, durable goods, pain management, case management, counseling, and social worker assistance. Routine intermittent home care must make up 80% of total care, with in-home continuous care and inpatient hospice care available for short periods.

68. B: All members of the interdisciplinary team (IDT) should be involved in developing the plan of care and in making major changes in the plan of care. However, individual members of the team may assume responsibility for more specific matters in which they are directly involved, such as titrating pain medication, skin care, and stress reduction. In many cases, the leader of the IDT is a physician, but decision-making should be a shared exercise. Nurses who provide direct care may have more insight into patient needs than other healthcare providers with less direct contact.

69. A: This is the accurate and appropriate answer. The Health Insurance Portability and Accountability Act (HIPAA) addresses the privacy of health information. It is essential to never release any information or documentation about a patient's condition or treatment without consent. Personal information about the patient is considered protected health information (PHI), and it includes any identifying or personal information about the patient, such as health history, condition, or treatments in any form, as well as any documentation. Failure to comply with HIPAA regulations can make one liable for legal action.

70. D: Excessive sleeping usually does not indicate pain. Careful observation of nonverbal behavior can indicate pain. These behaviors include:

- Respirations: Rapid and labored breathing increases as pain increases, with short periods of hyperventilation or Cheyne-Stokes respirations.
- Vocalization: Patient remains negative in speech or speaks quietly and reluctantly. Patient may moan or groan, call out, or cry.
- Facial expressions: Patient looks sad or frightened, frowning or grimacing, especially during activities that increase pain.
- Body language: Tense, fidgeting, pacing. As pain increases, patient may become rigid, clench fists, or lie in the fetal position and become increasingly combative.
- Consolability: Patient becomes less distractible or consolable.

71. D: While the patient has the legal right to make decisions, family and cultural dynamics vary widely, so pointing this out to the son or informing the patient of the issue may only cause conflict. A better approach is to arrange a family meeting with the son, the patient, and healthcare providers so that the patient can express opinions about who should make decisions, when it's appropriate for the son to make decisions, and what the patient ultimately wants. This is not an issue for the ethics committee.

72. C: Integrative outcomes data is particularly useful in evidence-based practice since it includes measures of mortality, longevity, and cost-effectiveness. A number of different types of outcomes data can also be considered:

- Clinical: Symptoms, diagnoses, staging of the disease, and indicators of individual health
- Physiological: Measures of physical abnormalities, loss of function, and activities of daily living
- Psychosocial: Feelings, perceptions, beliefs, functional impairment, and role performance
- Organizational: Readmissions, adverse reactions, and deaths

73. A: Some medications, such as codeine, may have pronounced side effects at doses high enough to be equianalgesic. Doses of codeine above 60 mg are not appropriate because the analgesic effect decreases with incrementally higher doses, and side effects (such as nausea, vomiting, and constipation) increase. When changing drugs, it's usually best to start at a dose that is slightly lower than the equianalgesic dose because tolerance to different drugs may vary.

74. B: In general, yes/no questions are easiest for patients with dysarthria. It's important not to rush patients or try to complete their statements for them. If the patient is not able to speak at all, then the patient's ability to indicate yes or no by blinking or nodding should be assessed. Dysarthria is unrelated to intelligence or hearing, so the nurse should use age-appropriate vocabulary and materials and speak in a normal tone of voice, facing the patient, so the nurse can observe gestures and facial expressions that the patient may use as augmentative and alternative communication (AAC).

75. C: The rescue dose for parenteral opioids should be approximately 25-50% of the hourly dose. Rescue doses are used as needed to relieve pain that breaks through despite regularly scheduled drugs. For patients on oral opioids, the rescue dose should be 5-15% of the 24-hour baseline dose. Rescue doses should be rapid-acting or immediate-release so that pain is controlled rapidly. The number of rescue doses needed in a 24-hour period helps to determine the need for titration of the baseline dose.

76. C: The most important consideration is the education and skills of the person to whom the task is delegated. The five rights of delegation include:

- Right task: Determine an appropriate task to delegate for a specific patient.
- Right circumstance: Consider the setting, resources, time factors, safety factors, and all other relevant information to determine the appropriateness of delegation.
- Right person: Choose the right person (by virtue of education and skills) to perform a task for the right patient.
- Right direction: Provide a clear description of the task, the purpose, any limits, and expected outcomes.
- Right supervision: Supervise, intervene as needed, and evaluate the performance of the task.

77. B: Sudden onset of confusion, restlessness, and anxiety in a dying patient is often caused by terminal delirium. This is common, affecting almost 90% of patients in the last one to two days of life. Pain usually decreases in the dying patient, so a severe, sudden increase in pain is not likely. A stroke would usually result in some evidence of weakness on one side, and the onset of symptoms with brain metastasis would be less abrupt. Medications, such as anti-anxiety agents (lorazepam) and neuroleptics (haloperidol) may relieve symptoms of delirium. Causes can include drug toxicity, distended bladder, or constipation.

78. A: Intravenous (IV) fluids may prolong dying rather than hastening death. Other disadvantages include an increased risk of:

- Congestive heart failure and pulmonary edema with increased dyspnea
- Skin breakdown due to increased urinary output and incontinence

On the other hand, providing IV fluids for hydration may relieve the family's anxiety that the patient is thirsty and may keep the mouth moist; educating family members about the dehydration in the death process may help allay this anxiety.

79. D: While all of these characteristics are important for team members, the willingness to compromise is central to collaboration. In addition, members must be able to communicate clearly, which encompasses assertiveness, patience, and empathy. Teams should identify specific challenges and problems and then focus on the task of reaching a solution. Collaboration is needed in order to move nursing forward. Nurses must take an active role in gathering data for evidence-based practice to support the role of nursing role in healthcare, and must share this information with other nurses and health professionals.

80. B: At death, pupils become fixed and dilated. Other indications of death include a lack of heartbeat and respirations. Body temperature begins to drop slowly, and the skin takes on a waxy pallor. The patient does not respond to stimuli. As the muscles relax, the patient may be incontinent of urine and/or feces. The dying process is generally not immediate, and these changes may not occur sequentially. For example, patients may stop breathing and then start again, or gasp several times, before breathing stops completely. Heartbeat should be assessed apically, as a weak pulse may not be evident peripherally.

81. A: Most patients who require increasing doses of opioids do so because their cancer is progressing, resulting in more pain. Addiction refers to compulsive use and cravings for drugs, and is rarely associated with pain treatment due to a life-threatening illness unless the patient had a prior addiction. Dependence refers to the need for a drug and resultant withdrawal effects if the drug is abruptly stopped or the dosage markedly lowered. Tolerance refers to the diminishing physiological response to a drug over time.

82. C: Pain in the right shoulder is a referred pain associated with liver cancer. As the cancer progresses, the liver enlarges, causing pain on the right side of the abdomen initially. The enlarging liver presses on nerves beneath the diaphragm, resulting in referred pain in the right shoulder. Liver cancer is often secondary to other cancers. However, when liver cancer is primary, the most common sites for metastasis are the lungs, portal veins, and regional lymph nodes.

83. D: Prealbumin (transthyretin) is most commonly monitored for acute changes in nutritional status because it has a half-life of only 2-3 days.

- Mild deficiency: 10-15 mg/dL
- Moderate deficiency: 5-9 mg/dL
- Severe deficiency: <5 mg/dL

Prealbumin is a good measurement because it quickly decreases when nutrition is inadequate and rises quickly in response to increased protein intake. Protein intake must be adequate to maintain levels of prealbumin. Total protein and transferrin levels can be influenced by many factors. Albumin has a half-life of 18-20 days, so it is sensitive to long-term protein deficiencies more than short-term.

84. B: Unless the family has explicitly asked not to be called, the family should be notified immediately that the patient's death is imminent so family members can be present if they wish. Usually only one person, such as a spouse, is notified, and that person notifies other family members. Death can be unpredictable, so if the patient is exhibiting signs of imminent death, then delaying the call may mean the family will not be there when the patient dies.

85. C: People may perceive and express pain differently, so unless drug-seeking or attention-seeking behavior has been established, the psychiatric or mental health nurse should accept the patient's pain as reported. Some cultures encourage outward expressions of pain while others do not. Various pain scales may be used, depending on the age and cognitive ability of the patient. The most commonly used scale for adolescents and adults is the 1-10 scale.

86. A: Many caregivers feel overwhelmed by their tasks and responsibilities, and voicing these feelings in a supportive group can be therapeutic. People in caregiver support groups also share strategies for coping with their problems. If no local program is available, online support groups may also be helpful. The daughter's statements reflect the reality of her situation and are not suggestive of depression, so a referral to a psychologist may not be necessary, though depression is common among caregivers. Arranging visits from a meals-on-wheels program may help to relieve some of the caregiver's burden. Friendly visitor programs vary but may allow the caregiver some brief periods of respite.

87. C: An effective strategy is to provide the patient with opportunities to make decisions; this can help the patient overcome feelings of uncertainty and help bolster confidence. Other strategies include providing companionship, listening, and encouraging the patient to express her feelings and concerns. Positive feedback and praise should only be given when appropriate to the situation. Telling the patient she has no reason to be depressed will invalidate her feelings and further lower her self-esteem. Low self-esteem is common among older adults because they have to deal with so many losses. They may become depressed, passive, and dependent.

88. D: Hospice benefits include short-term hospitalization for procedures such as pain control or for caregiver respite, but long-term hospitalization is not provided. Under current rules, hospice services can include physical therapy, occupational therapy, speech-language services, homemaker services, home health aide services, and durable medical supplies, such as hospital beds, commodes, dressing supplies, and disposable underwear. Medications and biologicals are also provided to hospice patients, as well as counseling services.

89. B: Willfully providing inadequate care while disregarding the safety and security of another is the definition of gross negligence. Negligence indicates that proper care has not been provided, based on established standards. Reasonable care is considered to be the decisions and processes that a reasonable health professional would generally follow when providing care. Gross negligence is the most serious kind of negligence, and signifies that the health professional acted recklessly and intentionally in failing to provide proper care. A less serious category of negligence is negligent conduct, which indicates that an individual failed to provide reasonable care or to protect or assist another, based on standards and expertise. Court cases involving negligence may consider contributory negligence as a factor if the injured party contributed in some way in causing the harm. Comparative negligence refers to an attempt to determine what percentage of the negligence can be attributed to each individual involved.

90. C: The legal document that designates someone to make decisions regarding medical and end-of-life care if a patient is mentally incompetent is known as a durable power of attorney. This is a type of advance directive, which can include living wills or specific patient requests regarding treatment. A "do not resuscitate" (DNR) order indicates that the patient does not want resuscitative treatment for any terminal illness or condition. A general power of attorney allows a designated person to make decisions for a person over broader areas, including financial matters.

91. A: Post-herpetic neuralgia is a chronic pain condition that responds poorly to opioids and is better treated with anticonvulsants, such as gabapentin. Tricyclic antidepressants are also used but may have severe side effects in elderly patients. Because the patient has been on high doses of hydrocodone, he may experience withdrawal with abrupt discontinuation of the drug, so the dose should be decreased by one tablet every 2-3 days, while gabapentin is started at a low dose and slowly increased, to reduce incidence of side effects. Morphine pumps and nonsteroidal anti-inflammatory drugs (NSAIDs) are usually avoided with warfarin and are often ineffective.

92. D: In most cases, careful observation of patients with Alzheimer's disease can help to determine what triggers agitation or outbursts so the triggers can be eliminated. When Alzheimer's patients receive too much input or feel overwhelmed, they may react negatively. Isolating the patient decreases social interaction and is rarely the answer. Making choices can be confusing and difficult, so asking patients to choose may increase agitation. Antipsychotic medications are generally contraindicated for Alzheimer's patients and do not attend to the underlying problem.

93. B: Chronic fatigue is usually associated with life-threatening illness and persists for more than 6 months. Acute or physiological fatigue has a specific cause and results in a general feeling of tiredness and impaired ability to carry out activities. Secondary fatigue results from pathology of disease processes and may relate to malnutrition, anemia, and side effects of medications. Peripheral fatigue results from impairment of the muscles, leading to instability.

94. A: While narcotic analgesia is an important component of pain management for advanced cervical cancer, bony metastasis usually responds best to radiation, which reduces pain. However, the patient may need to have 1-2 weeks of radiation treatment before experiencing any reduction in pain, so adjuvant therapy can be used to relieve pain in the interim period. Commonly used therapies include nonsteroidal anti-inflammatory drugs (NSAIDs) and tricyclic antidepressants, as well as other complementary therapies such as biofeedback, acupuncture, and massage. Radiation for pain management is acceptable for patients who are under hospice care.

95. C: Justice is the ethical principle that relates to the distribution of limited healthcare resources. These resources must be distributed fairly, and all parties involved should receive equal consideration. Making ethical and just decisions about limited resources can be difficult, but the nurse should consider which choice has optimum benefit for the greatest number of patients. Beneficence is an ethical precept stating that healthcare professionals should act in the best interests of their patients, while nonmaleficence is the ethical code of doing no harm. The autonomy of all patients—their right to make decisions about their treatment—is another aspect of medical ethics.

96. A: The anticholinergics glycopyrrolate and atropine are most commonly used to reduce bronchial death rattle. Both drugs can be administered subcutaneously and have rapid onset of action (about 1 minute); glycopyrrolate has a more potent effect. Morphine sulfate may reduce respiratory distress but does not generally affect death rales. The hyoscine hydrobromide (Scopolamine) transdermal patch has a slow onset of action (about 12 hours), so it is best used for long-term treatment. Oropharyngeal suctioning may relieve rales originating in the oropharynx but is ineffective for pooling of fluids in the bronchi.

97. B: Depression at the end of life is usually treated with selective serotonin reuptake inhibitors (SSRIs), although response may take a few weeks. Tricyclic antidepressants may have more adverse effects, and are contraindicated for older patients who are taking other medications. If life expectancy is very short, then stimulants such as dextroamphetamine are sometimes used to alleviate depression. For some depressed patients, psychotherapy may prove helpful as well. The cardinal signs of depression include mood changes, disturbances in perception, and behavioral changes. Dysphoria is common, and older adults may neglect personal hygiene and exhibit slow thought processes and withdrawal. Children may have somatic complaints. Grief and depression may present similarly, so a thorough interview is indicated.

98. B: The best approach to a life review is to ask open-ended questions such as "What is your earliest childhood memory?" to elicit information. While family members may participate, this is primarily an exercise to help the dying patient see the meaning in his or her own life. The nurse should start with questions about childhood and then move through the person's life periods chronologically, letting the patient guide the discussion as much as possible. Effective prompts include questions that ask the patient to assess his or her life: "Is there something you'd have done differently?" "How would you describe your life?"

99. A: The mother should be provided a quiet space and allowed to hold her child. In this early stage of grief, the mother may be overwhelmed and barely able to comprehend what has happened. While the other actions may be appropriate at some point, asking family members or a chaplain to intervene before the mother has had time to begin the grieving process, or listing hospital rules, may just increase the mother's stress.

100. D: When a medication has provided good pain control but significant side effects occur, the dose of the new opioid should start at 25-50% below the equianalgesic dose to try to avoid cross-tolerant symptoms. Rescue doses may be given with breakthrough pain. If the initial pain control was not adequate and significant side effects occurred, then opioids should be rotated at the equianalgesic dose. In either case, the patient must be monitored carefully for adverse effects.

101. C: Bereavement is the time period of mourning. This time period varies but may extend to a year or even longer. Grief is a normal response to loss, while mourning is the public expression of grief. There are three types of grief: acute, anticipatory, and chronic. Chronic grief is considered to be a serious risk and should be treated as depression, with antidepressants, psychological evaluation, and counseling. Depression is characterized by changes in mood and feelings of sadness.

102. B: Applying a pressure-reducing mattress or mattress overlay may help reduce friction and shear. Patients should be carefully positioned and supported, but comfort is the primary concern for dying patients. Avoiding pressure injuries is important, but in this case, changing the patient's position every two hours or lowering the head of the bed may result in more distress and discomfort, so the benefit may be negligible at best. Skin barriers should be routinely applied to the sacrococcygeal area.

103. C: "You are shaking and seem worried" acknowledges what is true and evident and leaves an opening for the patient to discuss his or her feelings if desired. "What's wrong?" requires a direct response that the patient may not feel like giving. "Do you want me to call your family?" does not deal with the patient's anxiety and is an escape for the nurse. "You don't need to worry. Everything will be all right" is a platitude that has little meaning and that may not, in fact, be true.

104. D: The nurse should attend to the spiritual needs of the patient by calling a priest even though the hour is not convenient. A Protestant chaplain cannot perform specific rituals that are important to many Catholic individuals, and the patient may not survive or be able to receive communion if the call is delayed. Catholic rituals include:

- Sacrament of the Anointing of the Sick: This replaces the last rites (Extreme Unction) and is a bedside blessing.
- *Viaticum*: This is essentially the last Holy Communion and is called the "food for the journey."

105. A: If the starting dose proves ineffective and the patient requires more than 4 rescue doses in 24 hours, the best action is to increase the baseline opioid dose. During titration, the dosage should be increased until optimal pain relief is achieved. Additionally, the rescue dosage should be increased along with the baseline dose so that they remain proportional. Generally, if one or two side effects occur, the medication is continued and side effects treated unless the side effects are severe. If more than two side effects occur, then opioid rotation may be indicated.

106. C: While all of these are important, patients who are homeless require further assistance with discharge, as compliance with treatment and follow-up appointments is poor in the homeless population. Interventions that are most important include:

- Lists of safe shelters and places they can go to bathe, eat, and get mail
- Help in applying for welfare assistance or Social Security

Discharge planning should begin on admission, and must be a joint effort, so that the transfer and discharge documents provide the information that the individual needs.

107. B: The minimal urinary output for an adult patient is 30 mL/hr, although this level cannot be sustained for long periods, as a more normal output is 40-60 mL/hr. Minimal output for an infant or child is 0.5 mL/kg/hr. Urinary output in an adult that is less than 30 mL/hr (or 0.5mL/kg/hr) may signal renal damage. Urinary output is influenced not only by renal status but also by hydration and medications. Vasoconstrictive medications may reduce urinary output. Patients may have low output after surgery, followed by diuresis, as their systems clear of anesthetic drugs and other medications.

108. C: Children should never be used as interpreters since they lack medical vocabulary and an understanding about health matters, and may not interpret correctly. Likewise, other adult family members (such as the wife) should not be asked to answer questions for the patient unless the patient is unable to answer questions because of a health condition, because they may not understand medical terms and may not translate correctly. Additionally, the patient may have kept information from the family.

109. B: The family should be encouraged to stay and talk to the patient, as hearing is usually the last of the senses to fail. Typical physical changes associated with death include:

- Sensory: Reduced sensations of pain and touch. Decreased vision and hearing.
- Circulatory: Tachycardia, followed by bradycardia; dysrhythmia; hypotension.
- Respiratory: Tachypnea progresses to Cheyne-Stokes respirations.
- Muscular: Muscles relax, jaw sags, and ability to swallow and talk is lost.
- Urinary: Output decreases, incontinence, and then anuria.
- Integumentary: Skin cold, clammy, cyanotic, and waxy. Coccygeal tear often occurs.

110. A: The Confusion Assessment Method is used to assess the development of delirium and is intended for use by those without psychiatric training. The assessment tool covers nine factors:

- Onset of acute changes in mental status
- Attention: Inattentive, stable, or fluctuating
- Thinking: Disorganized, rambling, switching topics, illogical
- Level of consciousness: Altered, ranging from alert to coma
- Orientation: Time, place, person
- Memory: Impairment
- Perceptual disturbances: Hallucinations, illusions
- Psychomotor abnormalities: Agitations or retardation
- Sleep-wake cycle: Awake at night, sleepy in daytime

Alzheimer's disease is assessed by a complete patient history, physical exam, and neurological exam. A determination of depression is also made. Substance abuse, including alcohol and prescription or nonprescription drugs, is assessed by a physical exam, patient interview, and use of screening tools such as the CAGE questions. Brain injuries are generally assessed by a neurological exam and imaging.

111. B: Moderately thickened liquids, such as split pea soup, are less likely to cause choking in patients with ALS than thin liquids, such as coffee. Products such as Thick-It are available to add to thin liquids, but infant rice cereal and yogurt may also be used. Foods that are sticky, such as white bread and thick oatmeal, may cause an obstructive plug to form. Finger foods, such as carrot sticks and hot dogs, may choke the patient if not chewed properly. The patient should be seated in upright position while eating. Providing a straw or sippy cup for liquids may help reduce choking.

112. C: The patient's estranged husband has been given a healthcare power of attorney, which gives him the right to make decisions if the patient is unable to do so. While divorce may automatically revoke the healthcare power of attorney in some states, the patient and her husband were not legally divorced. The legal document takes precedence over other family ties, such as those of the mother and daughter. This is not a decision that has to be rendered by an ethics committee. If family members want to challenge the husband, their recourse is to take the matter to court.

113. B: The patient is experiencing the denial stage of grief, during which a person may refuse to accept the diagnoses provided by doctors. People grieve differently and may not go through all five stages defined by Kübler-Ross's model, but most go through at least two of the stages. Kübler-Ross's five stages of grief are:

- Denial: Disbelieving, confused, stunned, detached, repeating questions
- Anger: Directed inward (self-blame) or outward
- Bargaining: If-then thinking (e.g., "If I go to church, then I will heal"); trying to find a different outcome
- Depression: Sad, withdrawn, tearful, crying, but beginning to accept loss
- Acceptance: Resolution and acceptance

114. A: Clouded consciousness is characterized by a general drowsy or sleepy appearance and inattention, although the patient can respond properly with persistence. Confusion can involve disorientation to time, person, place, or thing, as well as an inability to follow directions or difficulty doing so. Lethargy is characterized by more pronounced drowsiness. The patient may drift in and out of sleep, and some effort may be required to arouse the patient. Stupor is characterized by lack of responsiveness. The patient may be very difficult to arouse and usually lapses back into a stuporous state almost immediately after arousal.

115. D: Severe dehydration is fluid loss greater than 15%, and this occurs when total body water decreases but sodium does not. It is characterized by marked hypotension and anuria, as well as symptoms associated with lesser dehydration. Mild dehydration (5% loss) is characterized by dizziness, lethargy, reduced skin turgor, dry mucous membranes, and orthostatic hypotension. Moderate dehydration (10% loss) is characterized by confusion, resting hypotension, tachycardia, and oliguria/anuria. Dehydration may result from inadequate fluids, excess water loss, nasogastric suctioning, drugs, diarrhea, vomiting, or fever.

116. B: In almost all cases, pain control takes priority for dying patients because pain impacts all other areas. Patients in pain are often resistant to the moving or turning that is necessary to prevent pressure injuries, and may avoid eating or drinking, which affects nutrition and hydration. Comfort is more important than mobility in the late stages of dying, and controlling pain may allow the patient to be more mobile. Although one issue may have priority in a problem-focused care plan, different issues may be dealt with simultaneously.

117. A: Hyperkalemia (elevated levels of potassium in the blood) often occurs with renal disease and is characterized by ventricular arrhythmia, weakness with ascending paralysis and hyperreflexia, diarrhea, and confusion. Hypokalemia (reduced levels of potassium in the blood) is characterized by weakness, lethargy, nausea and vomiting, paresthesias, dysrhythmias (premature ventricular contractions, flattened T waves), muscle cramps with hyporeflexia, hypotension, and tetany. Hypocalcemia (reduced levels of calcium in the blood) is characterized by tetany, tingling, seizures, altered mental status, and ventricular tachycardia. Hypercalcemia (elevated levels of calcium in the blood) is characterized by increasing muscle weakness with hypotonicity, constipation, anorexia, nausea and vomiting, and bradycardia.

118. C: Hemorrhage of esophageal varices occurs in about a third of those with portal hypertension and is the most common cause of death with cirrhosis. As the portal vein becomes obstructed, increased pressure develops in vessels, especially in the lower esophagus and stomach, causing collateral vessels and varicosities to form. These collateral vessels are fragile and rupture easily. Jaundice, blockage of the bile duct, and Abdominal distension (ascites) occur with hepatic failure and are generally present before the development of portal hypertension.

119. C: Beck's triad is commonly found with cardiac tamponade. Other symptoms may include a feeling of pressure or pain in the chest, dyspnea, and pulsus paradoxus greater than 10 mmHg (systolic blood pressure heard during exhalation but not during inhalation). Cardiac tamponade occurs with pericardial effusion, in which fluid accumulates in the pericardial sac, causing pressure against the heart. It may be a complication of trauma, pericarditis, cardiac surgery, or heart failure.

120. D: Making a referral to a home health agency to provide in-home care is the best solution, as this ensures that the man will receive skilled nursing care and be able to stay at home with his grandson, who is too young for the responsibility of wound care. This is a more cost-effective solution than transferring the patient to an extended care facility. Keeping the patient in the hospital is generally not an option, as Medicare will not pay for extended care for long-term wound treatment.

121. B: Up to 30% of those who receive a peripheral neurolytic blockade may develop neuropathic pain because of inadequate denervation. Neural blockades can include peripheral blocks (cranial, brachial plexus, intercostal, and sacral), neuraxial (epidural/intrathecal), and sympathetic (celiac plexus, superior hypogastric). The adverse effects relate to the type and location of block. Adverse effects (such as numbness) may be temporary if a local anesthetic is used, or permanent if phenol or alcohol is used. Permanent neurological damage rarely occurs. Horner's syndrome, characterized by partial ptosis and miosis, can result from interscalene or supraclavicular blocks.

122. B: Pain medications are metabolized through the liver and excreted through the kidneys. As death nears and organ function decreases, the concentration of drug in the system increases, causing more sedation. The initial step should be to slowly decrease the dose to a level at which the patient remains comfortable but experiences less sedative effect. In some cases, if pain is severe, the dosage required to control pain results in inevitable sedation. Some patients who want to remain alert may refuse medication. In that case, alternative medications or methods of pain control may be tried.

123. C: Cordotomy is recommended for intractable unilateral pain below C-5 in patients whose life expectancy is less than one year. In some cases, pain on one side may be so severe that it masks pain on the other side, and this pain may become evident after the cordotomy. Additionally, while nociceptive pain may respond, neuropathic pain may not. Over time, pain may recur in some patients, and some will develop delayed post-cordotomy dysesthesia, making them sensitive to even benign stimuli.

124. D: While the patient's mood may be helpful in a pain diary, the essential elements include the name and dosage of the medication, the date and time the medication was taken, the intensity of pain prior to taking the medication, and the intensity of pain at a prescribed period after taking the medication (usually about 30 minutes for oral medications). Pain diaries are usually kept by the patients, allowing them to have some sense of control over their medications, but as the patient's condition deteriorates, caregivers may need to take over recording.

125. B: Music therapy should be tailored to the patient's preference, and this may vary from time to time. For example, a patient may prefer upbeat music during the daytime and quieter music in the evening. While soft classical music is a good general choice, some patients may prefer other genres. Some patients may favor music related to their culture. The delivery system may vary. In a single room, a radio or music player may be placed by the bed, but in a shared room, the volume should be turned down, or the patient should be fitted with small earphones.

126. C: Stage 3 lymphedema is usually characterized by unilateral non-pitting, hard edema from toes to groin, resulting from blockage of the lymph system. Lymphedema may also occur in the arms, especially for patients who have undergone mastectomy with removal of axillary lymph nodes. Most cases of lymphedema are secondary to a disease process (such as cancer) or treatment (such as radiation or surgery). Stage 1 lymphedema results in moderate swelling with slight pitting, while stage 2 involves fibrosis, with non-pitting but spongy tissue. Stage 3 lymphedema, also known as elephantiasis, involves severe swelling, huge enlargement of the involved extremity, and unresponsive fibrotic tissue.

127. A: Post-mastectomy pain syndrome (PMPS) is characterized by feelings of constriction, as well as burning, prickling, or numbness, primarily occurring in the posterior part of the arm on the affected side, the axillary region, or the chest wall. PMPS can occur following mastectomy with primary node dissection. Because movement increases pain, patients may be reluctant to move the arm on the affected side, sometimes resulting in a frozen shoulder. Treatment can include physical therapy and analgesia.

128. D: Deep, "squeezing" abdominal pain associated with nausea, vomiting, and diaphoresis is characteristic of visceral pain, which results from compression, swelling, or invasion of internal organs of the thorax or abdomen. When visceral pain is experienced in a part of the body away from the affected organ, it is classified as referred pain. Somatic pain is usually localized and relates to activation of pain sensors in the cutaneous and musculoskeletal tissues. Neuropathic pain is generally chronic and results from damage to the peripheral or central nervous systems.

129. B: Moderate anxiety is characterized by inattentiveness, narrow field of perception, and decreased observations. Mild anxiety is less noticeable, but patients have a decreased ability to solve problems and reduced awareness because attention is focusing inward. Severe anxiety is more obvious, as the patient may have outward expressions of anxiety, such as wringing the hands and wetting the lips; the patient's field of perception is limited. The patient is inattentive, and words and thoughts may seem scattered. Panic includes severe dread and fear, and is often accompanied by physical signs, such as chest pain, palpitations, and trembling. The patient has no field of perception.

130. D: Delirium is an acute sudden change in consciousness, characterized by reduced ability to focus or sustain attention, language and memory disturbance, disorientation, confusion, audiovisual hallucinations, sleep disturbance, and psychomotor activity disorder. Delirium differs from disorders with similar symptoms in that delirium is fluctuating, and symptoms tend to worsen at night. Delirium may result from drugs, such as anticholinergics, and numerous conditions, including infection, hypoxia, trauma, dementia, depression, vision and hearing loss, surgery, alcoholism, untreated pain, fluid/electrolyte imbalance, and malnutrition.

131. A: Hyperglycemia may result in sleepiness or stupor, as opposed to symptoms similar to anxiety. However, many conditions do present initially with symptoms similar to anxiety, and therefore may be overlooked or diagnosis delayed. Hypoxia can result in restlessness, tachypnea, lethargy, and poor judgment. Pulmonary embolus has similar symptoms, as well as chest pain, fever, and cough. Symptoms of an imbalance in electrolytes (such as sodium, calcium, and potassium) frequently include lethargy, irritability, and changes in mental status.

132. C: Changing to an equianalgesic may result in less drowsiness and lethargy, as patients may react differently to different drugs. Lowering the dose of medication will probably result in increased pain, and complementary therapies alone are rarely sufficient for severe pain. The patient always has the right to refuse medications, and insisting that the patient take the medication is a form of coercion. Patients may be willing to trade comfort for quality time with family or friends, but healthcare providers should seek alternatives.

133. B: A structured education plan for pain management should be presented to the patient after the pain has been controlled because the patient is less likely to comprehend the plan when in pain. Pain has a negative effect on cognition, and the anxiety associated with pain may also impact learning. Initially, the patient should be informed that the goal is to reduce pain. As the pain is controlled, the patient should receive education about the type of medication, dose, action, adverse effects, and managing breakthrough pain.

134. C: Distraction is most effective for short periods of discomfort, such as those associated with medical procedures. It is less effective for severe acute pain or chronic pain, although distraction may improve mood and relieve anxiety. Children are often distracted with toys, books, or games during procedures. A patient's interests should always be considered, since a distraction that does not interest someone is not effective. Distractions can be passive (e.g., watching television) or active (e.g., singing along with music or clapping hands).

135. C: Sodium should be restricted in the diet of a patient with ascites, as sodium can increase fluid retention. Canned and frozen foods should be avoided unless labeled "low sodium." Salt substitutes containing ammonia may cause hepatic coma and should be avoided. Patients with poor renal function should also avoid salt substitutes containing potassium. In most cases, diuretics are provided to prevent fluid retention. Patients often require education about foods and healthy eating, and encouragement to maintain a low-sodium diet.

136. D: The risk of gastrointestinal or central nervous system hemorrhage does not occur until the platelet count falls below 5,000 mm^3. A normal platelet count is 150,000 to 400,000 mm^3. Platelet counts below 50,000 mm^3 result in impaired clotting, and bleeding may occur with invasive procedures; however, risk is usually mild until the platelet count drops to below 20,000 mm^3, at which point petechiae, nasal and gingival bleeding, and excessive menstrual flow may occur. A decreased platelet count may result from reduced production of platelets, which can occur with leukemia and chemotherapy, and from increased destruction of platelets, which can occur with some diseases such as leukemia.

137. B: The patient should be offered food and fluids as long as the patient shows any interest. At some point, the patient may no longer want food or fluid or derive any pleasure from them, even though the patient may still be conscious. Lethargy does not warrant withholding food and fluids if the patient can be easily aroused from sleep. Artificial feeding and hydration is not recommended for patients who are dying because it extends suffering, although some patients and their families may choose this option.

138. A: While the patient's white blood count is within normal parameters, the normal absolute neutrophil count (ANC) for an adult is 1,800 to 7,700 mm^3. The risk of infection increases markedly if ANC falls below 1,000 mm^3 and is severe when ANC drops below 500 mm^3. A drop in ANC leads to neutropenia, a severe complication of chemotherapy and of some diseases, such as leukemia. Neutropenia increases the risk of both exogenous and endogenous infection. Patients with both neutropenia and a fever usually have an infection that could quickly become life-threatening.

139. D: Opioid-induced nausea and vomiting is best treated with haloperidol, which is also indicated when nausea and vomiting is triggered by anxiety. Scopolamine is indicated with intestinal obstruction, peritoneal irritation, and increased intracranial pressure. Metoclopramide relieves nausea and vomiting associated with gastric stasis, ileus, and chemotherapy. It is often also used to treat postoperative nausea and vomiting. Phenothiazines, including chlorpromazine and levomepromazine, are used for nausea and vomiting of unknown origin, intestinal obstruction, peritoneal irritation, increased intracranial pressure, and vestibular disturbances.

140. A: The lungs, liver, and bones are the most common sites for metastases. Some cancer cells migrate to other parts of the body but remain dormant, sometimes for a number of years, before growing. Any cancer can metastasize to any other part of the body, but many cancers preferentially metastasize to one or more sites.

Site of metastasis	Primary cancer
Lungs and liver	Breast, colon, kidney, lung, melanoma, ovary, pancreas, prostate, rectum, stomach, thyroid, and uterus
Bones	Breast, kidney, prostate, and thyroid
Peritoneum	Colon, ovary, pancreas, stomach, and uterus
Adrenal gland	Lung, rectum
Skin/muscle	Melanoma
Brain	Breast, colon, kidney, melanoma, and lung

141. B: Tasks should be completed slowly, sometimes broken into steps to be finished at intervals so the patient can rest in between. The patient should be positioned for comfort; positions may vary, but most people find that sitting with the head elevated, or even sitting upright and leaning slightly forward, relieves dyspnea to some degree. A cooling fan directing air toward the face can decrease the perception of dyspnea. If no fan is available, a patient may sit near an open window or air conditioning unit. Breathing exercises, such as pursed-lip and diaphragmatic breathing, may provide some relief.

142. C: The frequency of administration depends on the degree of pain and the type of medication. The goal of pain management is to avoid breakthrough pain, which can be debilitating and increase anxiety. Patients who are fearful of breakthrough pain may experience more pain because of anxiety. An important part of pain management is to anticipate adverse effects, such as constipation or sedation, and provide prophylaxis.

143. A: Octreotide, a somatostatin analog, is indicated for HIV/AIDS patients with secretory diarrhea. In some cases, anticholinergics, such as atropine or scopolamine, are also used. The drug of choice for treatment of diarrhea in patients in palliative care is loperamide (Imodium). Codeine, which has the side effect of constipation, can also be used to control diarrhea. Another choice is diphenoxylate (Lomotil). Loperamide and diphenoxylate should not be given to children under 12 and should be avoided with infectious diarrhea.

144. B: Dialysis is the best preventive method to relieve itching in patients with end-stage renal disease (ESRD). About 60% of patients with ESRD experience intense itching. Diet may be controlled to lower phosphorus intake. Treatments can include phosphate binders (calcium carbonate), activated vitamin D, antihistamines, urea, thalidomide, hydroxyzine, topical phenol solution, and corticosteroids. Phosphate binders may provide relief of itching, but may in turn cause gastric distention and nausea. Finding a treatment that relieves the patient's itching may require trial and error.

145. D: Jugular venous pressure (neck vein) is used to assess the cardiac output and pressure in the right heart, as the pulsations relate to changes in pressure in the right atrium. This procedure is usually not accurate if pulse rate is greater than 100. This is a noninvasive estimation of central venous pressure and waveform. Measurement should be done with the internal jugular if possible; if not, the external jugular may be used. Other signs of right-sided heart failure include decreased hemoglobin, peripheral edema, hepatosplenomegaly, and hepatojugular reflux. Daily weight gain is common.

146. C: An acute seizure is usually treated first with diazepam or lorazepam. If seizures persist, then phenytoin may be given with an intravenous loading dose for 24 hours followed by daily dosages to prevent recurrence of seizures. In some cases, phenobarbital may be used for long-term management. Corticosteroids may decrease intracranial pressure by reducing swelling around the tumor, thus reducing the risk of repeat seizures. Meperidine should be avoided in patients with seizures. The patient should be turned to the side during a seizure, and the body should be supported and protected, but the patient should not be restrained or have anything inserted into the mouth.

147. C: These symptoms are consistent with superior vena cava syndrome (SVCS), which can occur with invasion or compression of the superior vena cava. It is most commonly associated with lung cancer but can also occur with breast cancer, thymoma, and Kaposi's sarcoma. SVCS may result in cerebral anoxia, bronchial obstruction, or laryngeal edema unless promptly treated. Treatment can include radiation, chemotherapy, and surgery, but in a patient nearing death, supportive measures, such as oxygen therapy, corticosteroids, and diuretics, may relieve symptoms.

148. D: While hypnosis can bring about deep relaxation and help diminish perceptions of pain in some individuals, hypnosis requires focused concentration, and this can be difficult for patients who are weak, debilitated, or receiving opioids. Hypnosis is often achieved through imagery. Hypnotherapy should be carried out by trained professionals. Patients can learn techniques of self-hypnosis, as well, to relieve pain and dyspnea.

149. A: The patient should be in a sitting position, leaning onto a padded bedside stand, straddling a chair with the head supported on the back of the chair—or, if unable to sit, the patient should be lying on their side opposite the procedure site, with the head of the bed elevated 30-45° to ensure that fluid remains at the base. The patient should avoid coughing or moving during the procedure. A chest x-ray or ultrasound determines needle placement. After the procedure, the patient is monitored for cough, dyspnea, and hypoxemia.

150. B: These symptoms are consistent with obstruction of the small intestine. Sudden and frequent nausea and vomiting in large volumes, often immediately after intake, usually indicates a bowel obstruction in the small intestine, while obstructions of the colon usually result in more delayed vomiting, with fecal emesis. If obstruction is partial or inoperable, dexamethasone may relieve some of the symptoms because it reduces inflammation and swelling and provides relief of nausea.

It's Your Moment, Let's Celebrate It!

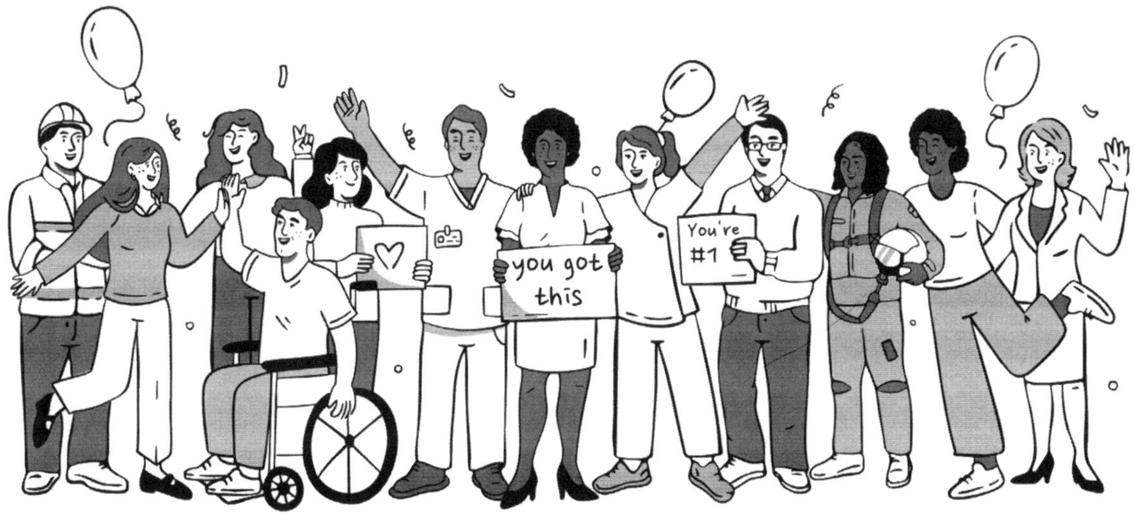

Share your story @mometrixtestpreparation